Exercise Evaluation and Prescription

Exercise Evaluation and Prescription

Editors

Cristina Cortis
Andrea Fusco
Carl Foster

MDPI • Basel • Beijing • Wuhan • Barcelona • Belgrade • Manchester • Tokyo • Cluj • Tianjin

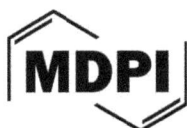

Editors

Cristina Cortis
Department of Human Sciences, Society and Health
University of Cassino and Lazio Meridionale
Cassino
Italy

Andrea Fusco
Department of Human Sciences, Society and Health
University of Cassino and Lazio Meridionale
Cassino
Italy

Carl Foster
Department of Exercise and Sport Science
University of Wisconsin-La Crosse
La Crosse
United States

Editorial Office
MDPI
St. Alban-Anlage 66
4052 Basel, Switzerland

This is a reprint of articles from the Special Issue published online in the open access journal *Journal of Functional Morphology and Kinesiology* (ISSN 2411-5142) (available at: www.mdpi.com/journal/jfmk/special_issues/Exercise_Evaluation).

For citation purposes, cite each article independently as indicated on the article page online and as indicated below:

LastName, A.A.; LastName, B.B.; LastName, C.C. Article Title. *Journal Name* **Year**, *Volume Number*, Page Range.

ISBN 978-3-0365-1384-3 (Hbk)
ISBN 978-3-0365-1383-6 (PDF)

© 2021 by the authors. Articles in this book are Open Access and distributed under the Creative Commons Attribution (CC BY) license, which allows users to download, copy and build upon published articles, as long as the author and publisher are properly credited, which ensures maximum dissemination and a wider impact of our publications.

The book as a whole is distributed by MDPI under the terms and conditions of the Creative Commons license CC BY-NC-ND.

Contents

About the Editors vii

Carl Foster, Cristina Cortis and Andrea Fusco
Exercise Evaluation and Prescription
Reprinted from: *Journal of Functional Morphology and Kinesiology* **2021**, 6, 31, doi:10.3390/jfmk6010031 1

Carl Foster, James D. Anholm, Daniel Bok, Daniel Boullosa, Giancarlo Condello, Cristina Cortis, Andrea Fusco, Salvador J. Jaime, Jos J. de Koning, Alejandro Lucia, John P. Porcari, Kim Radtke and Jose A. Rodriguez-Marroyo
Generalized Approach to Translating Exercise Tests and Prescribing Exercise
Reprinted from: *Journal of Functional Morphology and Kinesiology* **2020**, 5, 63, doi:10.3390/jfmk5030063 5

Thomas Gronwald, Alexander Törpel, Fabian Herold and Henning Budde
Perspective of Dose and Response for Individualized Physical Exercise and Training Prescription
Reprinted from: *Journal of Functional Morphology and Kinesiology* **2020**, 5, 48, doi:10.3390/jfmk5030048 15

Roberto Pippi, Andrea Di Blasio, Cristina Aiello, Carmine Fanelli, Valentina Bullo, Stefano Gobbo, Lucia Cugusi and Marco Bergamin
Effects of a Supervised Nordic Walking Program on Obese Adults with and without Type 2 Diabetes: The C.U.R.I.A.Mo. Centre Experience
Reprinted from: *Journal of Functional Morphology and Kinesiology* **2020**, 5, 62, doi:10.3390/jfmk5030062 23

Francesco Campa, Pasqualino Maietta Latessa, Gianpiero Greco, Mario Mauro, Paolo Mazzuca, Federico Spiga and Stefania Toselli
Effects of Different Resistance Training Frequencies on Body Composition, Cardiometabolic Risk Factors, and Handgrip Strength in Overweight and Obese Women: A Randomized Controlled Trial
Reprinted from: *Journal of Functional Morphology and Kinesiology* **2020**, 5, 51, doi:10.3390/jfmk5030051 37

Ulric S. Abonie, Femke Hoekstra, Bregje L. Seves, Lucas H. V. van der Woude, Rienk Dekker and Florentina J. Hettinga
Associations between Activity Pacing, Fatigue, and Physical Activity in Adults with Multiple Sclerosis: A Cross Sectional Study
Reprinted from: *Journal of Functional Morphology and Kinesiology* **2020**, 5, 43, doi:10.3390/jfmk5020043 49

Gabriele Mascherini, Benedetta Tosi, Chiara Giannelli, Elena Ermini, Leonardo Osti and Giorgio Galanti
Adjuvant Therapy Reduces Fat Mass Loss during Exercise Prescription in Breast Cancer Survivors
Reprinted from: *Journal of Functional Morphology and Kinesiology* **2020**, 5, 49, doi:10.3390/jfmk5030049 59

Grazia Maugeri and Giuseppe Musumeci
Adapted Physical Activity to Ensure the Physical and Psychological Well-Being of COVID-19 Patients
Reprinted from: *Journal of Functional Morphology and Kinesiology* **2021**, 6, 13, doi:10.3390/jfmk6010013 . . . . **69**

Meghan K. Magee, Brittanie L. Lockard, Hannah A. Zabriskie, Alexis Q. Schaefer, Joel A. Luedke, Jacob L. Erickson, Margaret T. Jones and Andrew R. Jagim
Prevalence of Low Energy Availability in Collegiate Women Soccer Athletes
Reprinted from: *Journal of Functional Morphology and Kinesiology* **2020**, 5, 96, doi:10.3390/jfmk5040096 . . . . **77**

Alexandros Savvides, Christoforos D. Giannaki, Angelos Vlahoyiannis, Pinelopi S. Stavrinou and George Aphamis
Effects of Dehydration on Archery Performance, Subjective Feelings and Heart Rate during a Competition Simulation
Reprinted from: *Journal of Functional Morphology and Kinesiology* **2020**, 5, 67, doi:10.3390/jfmk5030067 . . . . **87**

Tindaro Bongiovanni, Gabriele Mascherini, Federico Genovesi, Giulio Pasta, Fedon Marcello Iaia, Athos Trecroci, Marco Ventimiglia, Giampietro Alberti and Francesco Campa
Bioimpedance Vector References Need to Be Period-Specific for Assessing Body Composition and Cellular Health in Elite Soccer Players: A Brief Report
Reprinted from: *Journal of Functional Morphology and Kinesiology* **2020**, 5, 73, doi:10.3390/jfmk5040073 . . . . **97**

Cristian Petri, Francesco Campa, Vitor Hugo Teixeira, Pascal Izzicupo, Giorgio Galanti, Angelo Pizzi, Georgian Badicu and Gabriele Mascherini
Body Fat Assessment in International Elite Soccer Referees
Reprinted from: *Journal of Functional Morphology and Kinesiology* **2020**, 5, 38, doi:10.3390/jfmk5020038 . . . . **105**

Daniel Rojas-Valverde, Rafael Timón, Braulio Sánchez-Ureña, José Pino-Ortega, Ismael Martínez-Guardado and Guillermo Olcina
Potential Use of Wearable Sensors to Assess Cumulative Kidney Trauma in Endurance Off-Road Running
Reprinted from: *Journal of Functional Morphology and Kinesiology* **2020**, 5, 93, doi:10.3390/jfmk5040093 . . . . **115**

Felice Sirico, Veronica Romano, Anna Maria Sacco, Immacolata Belviso, Vittoria Didonna, Daria Nurzynska, Clotilde Castaldo, Stefano Palermi, Giuseppe Sannino, Elisabetta Della Valle, Stefania Montagnani and Franca Di Meglio
Effect of Video Observation and Motor Imagery on Simple Reaction Time in Cadet Pilots
Reprinted from: *Journal of Functional Morphology and Kinesiology* **2020**, 5, 89, doi:10.3390/jfmk5040089 . . . . **125**

Brooke V. Harmon, Andrea N. Reed, Rebecca R. Rogers, Mallory R. Marshall, Joseph A. Pederson, Tyler D. Williams and Christopher G. Ballmann
Differences in Balance Ability and Motor Control between Dancers and Non-Dancers with Varying Foot Positions
Reprinted from: *Journal of Functional Morphology and Kinesiology* **2020**, 5, 54, doi:10.3390/jfmk5030054 . . . . **135**

About the Editors

Cristina Cortis

Cristina Cortis is currently Associate Professor in Sports Science at the Department of Human Sciences, Society and Health, at the University of Cassino and Lazio Meridionale, Italy. She obtained a PhD degree in 2009 in Sport and Health Sciences at the University of Rome "Foro Italico", Italy. She was Visiting Researcher at the Human Performance Laboratory of the University of Wisconsin La Crosse (USA) and University of Connecticut (USA). Prof. Dr. Cortis has been recognized as a Fellow of the American College of Sports Medicine in 2020.

Andrea Fusco

Andrea Fusco is currently a post-doc researcher and Lecturer in Sport Science at the Department of Human Sciences, Society and Health at the University of Cassino and Lazio Meridionale, Italy. He obtained a Ph.D. degree in the field of Sport and Health Sciences at the University of Cassino and Lazio Meridionale, Italy, receiving the title of Doctor Europaeus. He was also visiting researcher at the Human Performance Laboratory of the University of Wisconsin La Crosse (USA) and Biomechanics Laboratory at the Department of Sport Science and Kinesiology of the University of Salzburg (Austria).

Carl Foster

Carl Foster is a Professor Emeritus in Exercise and Sports Science at the University of Wisconsin-La Crosse. He received his Ph.D. (1976) from the University of Texas at Austin. From 1977 to 1998, he was Professor of Medicine in the University of Wisconsin-Medical School at Sinai Samaritan Medical Center in Milwaukee, after which he moved to UW-La Crosse. He is a Fellow of ACSM and AACVPR, and has been President (2005-2006) and Treasurer (2015-2021) of ACSM. He received the Citation Award from ACSM (2009) and the ML Pollock Established Investigator Award from AACVPR (2010). From 1989 to 2003 he was an Associate Editor of Medicine and Science in Sports and Exercise, and, from 2009 to 2013, he was Editor-in-Chief of the International Journal of Sports Physiology and Performance. From 1983 to 2002, he was the chair of the Sports Medicine and Sports Science Committee of U.S. Speed Skating.

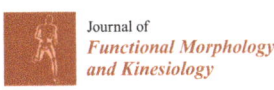

Editorial
Exercise Evaluation and Prescription

Carl Foster [1], Cristina Cortis [2,*] and Andrea Fusco [2,*]

1. Department of Exercise and Sport Science, University of Wisconsin-La Crosse, La Crosse, WI 54601, USA; cfoster@uwlax.edu
2. Department of Human Sciences, Society and Health, University of Cassino and Lazio Meridionale, 03043 Cassino, Italy
* Correspondence: c.cortis@unicas.it (C.C.); andrea.fusco@unicas.it (A.F.)

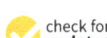

Citation: Foster, C.; Cortis, C.; Fusco, A. Exercise Evaluation and Prescription. *J. Funct. Morphol. Kinesiol.* 2021, 6, 31. https://doi.org/10.3390/jfmk6010031

Received: 3 March 2021
Accepted: 19 March 2021
Published: 23 March 2021

Publisher's Note: MDPI stays neutral with regard to jurisdictional claims in published maps and institutional affiliations.

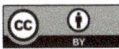

Copyright: © 2021 by the authors. Licensee MDPI, Basel, Switzerland. This article is an open access article distributed under the terms and conditions of the Creative Commons Attribution (CC BY) license (https://creativecommons.org/licenses/by/4.0/).

Ever since the farm boy, Milo of Crotone, lifted a growing bullock every day, to become the strongest man in the world, and six-time champion of the ancient Olympic Games, we have known about the principle of progression of exercise training. Probably earlier, but certainly by the early 1950's, Matti Karvonen in Finland [1] taught us that there was a minimal intensity of exercise training necessary to provoke a training response. Thus, we learned that prescription of training was based on an evaluation of the potential exerciser, in order to pick an appropriate relative training intensity [2]. Evaluative procedures that are highly individually specific are critical. By the mid 1970's, several investigators demonstrated that various combinations of training frequency, intensity, type and training time (FITT) could produce predictable results in exercise capacity. This extensive body of knowledge is codified in documents like ACSM's Guidelines for Exercise Testing and Prescription, now in its' 10th edition [3].

Although training intensity and duration were originally based on the relative percent concept of Karvonen, more contemporary approaches have emphasized threshold-based prescription [4], and on simple psychophysiological approaches like rating of perceived exertion [5] and the Talk Test [6]. These latter approaches are somewhat evaluation independent in terms of prescribing the training load, but evaluation is still important in terms of assessing the outcomes of training.

Sometime in the intervening years, we learned about the concept of a "therapeutic window", the dynamic space between the good effects and bad side-effects, such as myocardial infarction, that come from exercise training programs. We also learned about the interplay between the fitness that increases with training and the fatigue (often a precursor to injury) that comes with the same training program. This interplay is the nucleus of the training impulse (TRIMP) concept of Banister [7], which essentially underpins monitoring training programs. Within this space lies the business of exercise prescription. In athletes, operating outside the therapeutic window is likely to cause injuries that interfere with the goals of the training program. If they cause an athlete to miss important competitions, they can be quite meaningful, but are rarely permanent or life threatening. However, given the social and financial importance of contemporary high-level sport, missing such competitions simply because athletes ignored common sense advice is unreasonable. In the ever-increasing population of older exercisers, or of patients where exercise is part of a rehabilitation program, side effects can be more severe, often life threatening, although predictable and manageable [8]. Thus, understanding the parameters of the therapeutic window is critical to successful prescription of training programs.

This volume presents several papers, written from the perspective of optimizing training programs by better understanding the purpose and process of evaluating exercise capacity either in order to better prescribe exercise training or to better understand the outcome of exercise training programs. A total of 14 papers were published, including nine original articles, two viewpoints, two brief reports, and a review, focusing on healthy and sport population (soccer, off-road running, archery, dance, and pilot cadets) and diseases (type II diabetes, overweight, obese, breast cancer survivors, multiple sclerosis, and COVID-19 patients).

In order to carefully adjust training intensity and duration prescription, Foster et al. [9] suggested the utility of "translating" exercise test responses into the workload during exercise training. In particular, in sedentary individuals beginning an exercise program or in patients during rehabilitation, this approach may yield useful estimates of exercise intensity and contribute to both the safety and efficacy of exercise therapy. Accordingly, to implement physical interventions effectively, it is essential to provide an appropriate exercise and training prescription terminology. Therefore, Gronwald et al. [10] provided a new and clearer definition of the terms dose and response in the context of exercise and training prescription, suggesting that the dose of physical exercise and/or physical training should be operationalized by specific markers of internal load and modifying the exercise prescription by carefully adjusting the external load.

Individualized and supervised training FITT prescription are particularly important for specific clinical populations and in particular situations such as the health-related consequences of COVID-19. In fact, Pippi et al. [11] with the C.U.R.I.A.Mo. Centre Experience showed the effectiveness and the importance of a supervised Nordic walk program to improve body weight control, body composition parameters, muscular flexibility and maximal oxygen uptake levels in obese adults with and without type 2 diabetes. Furthermore, Campa et al. [12] showed that a supervised high frequency resistance training program resulted in greater benefits for weight loss, cardiometabolic risk factors and handgrip strength than a training program with a session once a week in overweight and obese women. Additionally, the lack of significant associations between activity pacing and fatigue or physical activity found by Abonie et al. [13] suggests that people with multiple sclerosis which may benefit from targeted interventions to manage fatigue and optimize engagement in physical activity. Mascherini et al. [14] demonstrated that an exercise prescription program produces mid-term improvements in body composition, physical fitness and health-related quality of life of breast cancer survivors while adjuvant therapy slows down the effectiveness of an exercise program in the loss of fat mass. Individualization and personalization are also the key terms of the review proposed by Maugeri and Musumeci [15]. Accordingly, they provided a detailed review of the literature aiming to summarize updated evidence on the beneficial effects of adapted physical activity, based on personalized and tailor-made exercise, in preventing, treating, and counteracting the consequences of COVID-19.

The dose–response relationship proposed by Gronwald et al. [10] depends on a multitude of factors, such as internal and external load, and influencing factors. Within the influencing factors, nutrition, hydration, anthropometrics, environment, sport specific circumstances and ability have been highlighted. Results from Magee et al. [16] demonstrated a continued need for sport nutrition education interventions to be part of regular team activities, recommended to help athletes understand their advanced dietary requirements, provide strategies to meet dietary recommendations and avoid low energy availability. Investigating the effect of dehydration on archery performance, subjective feelings and heart rate response, the study from Savvides et al. [17] reported that, despite the induced psychological and physiological strain, archery performance over 72 arrows was not affected by dehydration. Specific bioelectrical impedance vector analysis references for the start of the season period, through which the physical condition achieved after the preparation microcycle in soccer can be assessed, have been provided by Bongiovanni et al. [18]. Thanks to findings from Petri et al. [19], national and international federations will be able to perform regular body composition assessments using skinfold measurements in soccer referees. Rojas-Valverde et al. [20] showed that data related to impacts could better explain the cumulative mechanical kidney trauma during mountain running, suggesting technology to better understand how the number and magnitude of the g-forces involved in off-road running could potentially affect kidney function. Video observation and motor imagery training did not improve reaction time when compared to controls, but Sirico et al. [21] suggested it as a useful training strategy in individuals who need to simultaneously develop a fast response to different types of stimuli like pilot cadets. Finally, dance participation and experience proved to not influence balance and motor control in the sixth ballet position although resulting in better balance outcomes while standing in the first ballet position, suggesting identifying specific training adaptations and injury risk in varying foot positions [22].

Given the great success of the present Special Issue, we already launched a second edition, and we do hope to receive contributions focusing on the use of either laboratory or field evaluations to generate training advice in patients, healthy people, and athletes.

Funding: This research received no external funding.

Conflicts of Interest: The authors declare no conflict of interest.

References

1. Karvonen, M.; Kentala, E.; Mustala, O. The effects of training on heart rate; a longitudinal study. *Ann. Med. Exp. Biol. Fenn* **1957**, *35*, 307–315. [PubMed]
2. Impellizzeri, F.M.; Marcora, S.M.; Coutts, A.J. Internal and external training load: 15 years on. *Int. J. Sports Physiol. Perform.* **2019**, *14*, 270–273. [CrossRef] [PubMed]
3. American College of Sports Medicine. *ACSM's Guidelines for Exercise Testing and Prescription*, 10th ed.; Wolters Kluwer: Alphen aan den Rijn, The Netherlands, 2017; ISBN 9788578110796.
4. Mezzani, A.; Hamm, L.F.; Jones, A.M.; McBride, P.E.; Moholdt, T.; Stone, J.A.; Urhausen, A.; Williams, M.A. Aerobic Exercise Intensity Assessment and Prescription in Cardiac Rehabilitation. *J. Cardiopulm. Rehabil. Prev.* **2012**, *32*, 327–350. [CrossRef] [PubMed]
5. Foster, C.; Boullosa, D.; McGuigan, M.; Fusco, A.; Cortis, C.; Arney, B.E.; Orton, B.; Jaime, S.J.; Radtke, K.; van Erp, T.; et al. 25 years of session RPE: Historical perspective and development. *Int. J. Sports Physiol. Perform.* **2021**, in press.
6. Foster, C.; Porcari, J.P.; Doro, K.; Dubiel, J.; Engen, M.; Kolman, D.; Ault, S.; Xiong, S. Exercise prescription when there is no exercise test: The Talk Test. *Kinesiology* **2018**, *50*, 333–348.
7. Banister, E.W. Modeling elite athletic performance. In *Physiological Testing of Elite Athletes*; Green, H., McDougal, J., Wenger, H., Eds.; Human Kinetics: Champaign, IL, USA, 1991; pp. 403–424.
8. Foster, C.; Porcari, J.P.; Battista, R.A.; Udermann, B.; Wright, G.; Lucia, A. The Risk in Exercise Training. *Am. J. Lifestyle Med.* **2008**, *2*, 279–284. [CrossRef]
9. Foster, C.; Anholm, J.D.; Bok, D.; Boullosa, D.; Condello, G.; Cortis, C.; Fusco, A.; Jaime, S.J.; de Koning, J.J.; Lucia, A.; et al. Generalized approach to translating exercise tests and prescribing exercise. *J. Funct. Morphol. Kinesiol.* **2020**, *5*, 63. [CrossRef]
10. Gronwald, T.; Törpel, A.; Herold, F.; Budde, H. Perspective of dose and response for individualized physical exercise and training prescription. *J. Funct. Morphol. Kinesiol.* **2020**, *5*, 48. [CrossRef]
11. Pippi, R.; Di Blasio, A.; Aiello, C.; Fanelli, C.; Bullo, V.; Gobbo, S.; Cugusi, L.; Bergamin, M. Effects of a supervised nordic walking program on obese adults with and without type 2 diabetes: The C.U.R.I.A.Mo. Centre experience. *J. Funct. Morphol. Kinesiol.* **2020**, *5*. [CrossRef]
12. Campa, F.; Latessa, P.M.; Greco, G.; Mauro, M.; Mazzuca, P.; Spiga, F.; Toselli, S. Effects of different resistance training frequencies on body composition, cardiometabolic risk factors, and handgrip strength in overweight and obese women: A randomized controlled trial. *J. Funct. Morphol. Kinesiol.* **2020**, *5*, 1–12. [CrossRef] [PubMed]
13. Abonie, U.S.; Hoekstra, F.; Seves, B.L.; Van Der Woude, L.H.V.; Dekker, R.; Hettinga, F.J. Associations between activity pacing, fatigue, and physical activity in adults with multiple sclerosis: A cross sectional study. *J. Funct. Morphol. Kinesiol.* **2020**, *5*, 43. [CrossRef] [PubMed]
14. Mascherini, G.; Tosi, B.; Giannelli, C.; Ermini, E.; Osti, L.; Galanti, G. Adjuvant therapy reduces fat mass loss during exercise prescription in breast cancer survivors. *J. Funct. Morphol. Kinesiol.* **2020**, *5*, 49. [CrossRef] [PubMed]
15. Maugeri, G.; Musumeci, G. Adapted Physical Activity to Ensure the Physical and Psychological Well-Being of COVID-19 Patients. *J. Funct. Morphol. Kinesiol.* **2021**, *6*, 13. [CrossRef] [PubMed]
16. Magee, M.K.; Lockard, B.L.; Zabriskie, H.A.; Schaefer, A.Q.; Luedke, J.A.; Erickson, J.L.; Jones, M.T.; Jagim, A.R. Prevalence of Low Energy Availability in Collegiate Women Soccer Athletes. *J. Funct. Morphol. Kinesiol.* **2020**, *5*, 96. [CrossRef] [PubMed]
17. Savvides, A.D.; Giannaki, C.; Vlahoyiannis, A.S.; Stavrinou, P.; Aphamis, G. Effects of Dehydration on Archery Performance, Subjective Feelings and Heart Rate during a Competition Simulation. *J. Funct. Morphol. Kinesiol.* **2020**, *5*, 67. [CrossRef] [PubMed]
18. Bongiovanni, T.; Mascherini, G.; Genovesi, F.; Pasta, G.; Iaia, F.M.; Trecroci, A.; Ventimiglia, M.; Alberti, G.; Campa, F. Bioimpedance vector references need to be period-specific for assessing body composition and cellular health in elite soccer players: A brief report. *J. Funct. Morphol. Kinesiol.* **2020**, *5*, 73. [CrossRef] [PubMed]
19. Petri, C.; Campa, F.; Teixeira, V.H.; Izzicupo, P.; Galanti, G.; Pizzi, A.; Badicu, G.; Mascherini, G. Body fat assessment in international elite soccer referees. *J. Funct. Morphol. Kinesiol.* **2020**, *5*, 38. [CrossRef] [PubMed]

20. Rojas-Valverde, D.; Timón, R.; Sánchez-Ureña, B.; Pino-Ortega, J.; Martínez-Guardado, I.; Olcina, G. Potential Use of Wearable Sensors to Assess Cumulative Kidney Trauma in Endurance Off-Road Running. *J. Funct. Morphol. Kinesiol.* **2020**, *5*, 93. [CrossRef] [PubMed]
21. Sirico, F.; Romano, V.; Sacco, A.M.; Belviso, I.; Didonna, V.; Nurzynska, D.; Castaldo, C.; Palermi, S.; Sannino, G.; Della Valle, E.; et al. Effect of Video Observation and Motor Imagery on Simple Reaction Time in Cadet Pilots. *J. Funct. Morphol. Kinesiol.* **2020**, *5*, 89. [CrossRef] [PubMed]
22. Harmon, B.V.; Reed, A.N.; Rogers, R.R.; Marshall, M.R.; Pederson, J.A.; Williams, T.D.; Ballmann, C.G. Differences in balance ability and motor control between dancers and non-dancers with varying foot positions. *J. Funct. Morphol. Kinesiol.* **2020**, *5*, 54. [CrossRef] [PubMed]

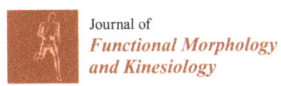

Viewpoint

Generalized Approach to Translating Exercise Tests and Prescribing Exercise

Carl Foster [1,*], James D. Anholm [2], Daniel Bok [3], Daniel Boullosa [4,5], Giancarlo Condello [6], Cristina Cortis [7], Andrea Fusco [7], Salvador J. Jaime [1], Jos J. de Koning [1,8], Alejandro Lucia [9,10], John P. Porcari [1], Kim Radtke [1] and Jose A. Rodriguez-Marroyo [11]

1. Department of Exercise and Sport Science, University of Wisconsin-La Crosse, La Crosse, WI 54601, USA; sjaime@uwlax.edu (S.J.J.); j.j.de.koning@vu.nl (J.J.d.K.); jporcari@uwlax.edu (J.P.P.); kradtke@uwlax.edu (K.R.)
2. VA Medical Health Care System, Loma Linda, CA 92697, USA; James.Anholm@va.gov
3. Faculty of Kinesiology, University of Zagreb, 10000 Zagreb, Croatia; daniel.bok@kif.unizg.hr
4. INISA, Federal University of Mato Grosso do Sul, Campo Grande 79070-900, Brazil; daniel.boullosa@gmail.com
5. College of Healthcare Sciences, James Cook University, Townsville 4811, Australia
6. Graduate Institute of Sports Training, Institute of Sports Sciences, University of Taipei, Taipei 111, Taiwan; giancarlo.condello@gmail.com
7. Department of Human Sciences, Society and Health, University of Cassino and Lazio Meridionale, 03043 Cassino, Italy; c.cortis@unicas.it (C.C.); andrea.fusco@unicas.it (A.F.)
8. Department of Human Movement Science, Movement Sciences Amsterdam, Vrije Universiteit, 1081BT Amsterdam, The Netherlands
9. Faculty of Sport Sciences, Universidad Europea de Madrid, 28670 Villaviciosa de Odón, Spain; alejandro.lucia@universidadeuropea.es
10. Research Institute 'imas12', Hospital 12 de Octubre, 28041 Madrid, Spain
11. Department of Physical Education and Sports, University of León, 24071 León, Spain; j.marroyo@unileon.es
* Correspondence: cfoster@uwlax.edu

Received: 11 July 2020; Accepted: 10 August 2020; Published: 12 August 2020

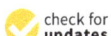

Abstract: Although there is evidence supporting the benefit of regular exercise, and recommendations about exercise and physical activity, the process of individually prescribing exercise following exercise testing is more difficult. Guidelines like % heart rate (HR) reserve (HRR) require an anchoring maximal test and do not always provide a homogenous training experience. When prescribing HR on the basis of % HRR, rating of perceived exertion or Talk Test, cardiovascular/perceptual drift during sustained exercise makes prescription of the actual workload difficult. To overcome this issue, we have demonstrated a strategy for "translating" exercise test responses to steady state exercise training on the basis of % HRR or the Talk Test that appeared adequate for individuals ranging from cardiac patients to athletes. However, these methods depended on the nature of the exercise test details. In this viewpoint, we combine these data with workload expressed as Metabolic Equivalent Task (METs). We demonstrate that there is a regular stepdown between the METs during training to achieve the same degree of homeostatic disturbance during testing. The relationship was linear, was highly-correlated (r = 0.89), and averaged 71.8% (Training METs/Test METs). We conclude that it appears possible to generate a generalized approach to correctly translate exercise test responses to exercise training.

Keywords: exercise prescription; target heart rate; RPE; Talk Test

1. Introduction

Exercise is a very positive health behavior. As far back as Hippocrates in the 4th century Before Common Era (BCE) and Galen in the 3rd century BCE, the concept of *mens sana in corpore sano* "a healthy mind in a healthy body" has been one of the cornerstones of medical practice. Exercise is particularly beneficial considering that in most of the developed world, heart disease is the leading attributable cause of death (45–50% of deaths), and cancer the 2nd (30–35% of deaths), although their incidence is meaningfully reduced in people who follow out genetic heritage and perform a large volume of exercise [1]. Despite the development of significant diagnostic and therapeutic medical options, the incidence of both diseases rose steadily through the first 70 years of the 20th century and began to decline after the 1962 publication of the United States Surgeon General's recommendations against smoking [2] and Cooper's Aerobics in 1968 [3], which essentially launched the "jogging" movement. The evidence supporting the positive health benefit of regular exercise is based on an abundant data base of epidemiological studies [4–8]. More recent population studies have demonstrated a dose–response effect of exercise on the risk of mortality, with an apparent saturation of benefit at ~20 Metabolic Equivalent Task (MET) hours per week [9–14]. There is, paradoxically, a slight excess in mortality above ~75 MET hours per week [9–11]. This is paralleled by a progressive reduction in the probability of cardiovascular events with increases in the number of steps accumulated per day [12–14].

Table 1. Negative outcomes during exercise training.

Congenital Abnormalities
Hypertrophic cardiomyopathy
Arrhythmogenic RV dysplasia
Coronary artery anomalies
Undiagnosed Coronary Artery Disease
Pre-exercise screening identifies >50%
First presentation of cardiovascular disease is often fatal 33% males, 12% females
Drug Use
Anabolic steroids
Stimulants
Erythropoietin
Recreational drugs
Trauma
Commotio cordis

With any health/medical therapy, particularly with drugs and surgery, there are usually iatrogenic (negative) side effects that need to be accounted for, which influences the dose of exercise recommended. In the 19th century, exercise (particularly athletics) was often viewed with some suspicion [15–17]. A series of reports, based on data collected after the beginning of the "jogging revolution" following the 1968 publication of Cooper's Aerobics, suggested that middle-aged joggers were at somewhat of an increased risk during exercise [17]. This risk was largely seen to be based on a changed flow–demand relationship in the coronary circulation and the risk of rupturing of existing atherosclerotic plaque. Negative outcomes during exercise training appear to be based on a variety of factors (Table 1) [18]. In adults, early studies suggested that bad outcomes during exercise were most often seen in persons with underling coronary artery disease [17], and that the presentation of myocardial infarction vs. sudden cardiac death seemed to be related to the presence/absence of prior myocardial infarction (e.g., prior myocardial scarring) [17]. In the 1990s, a series of studies focused on the "triggering" of myocardial infarction, noted that when exercise was involved, it was usually "unaccustomed heavy (>6 METs) exercise" in previously sedentary individuals" [17]. Across time, the risk of untoward events during exercise training, whether in healthy individuals or patients with known cardiovascular disease, has generally decreased [15], perhaps largely because we have become better at recognizing when not to begin an exercise program, and by recognizing the importance of controlling intensity during the early days/weeks of an exercise program [15].

2. Exercise Testing

Graded exercise testing is a fundamental technique within medical diagnostics, fitness assessment, performance diagnostics, and exercise prescription [18–20]. There are a variety of reasons for exercise testing (Table 2) [18]. Exercise testing, which at the minimum usually involves progressively harder exercise, with electrocardiogram (ECG) and hemodynamic monitoring, can be augmented in a variety of ways including measurement of respiratory gas exchange, and methods designed to measure myocardial perfusion or ventricular function [19]. Exercise capacity derived from graded exercise tests has been shown to be very useful in terms of defining prognosis [21,22]. In middle-aged individuals, including patients with known cardiovascular disease, peak exercise capacities of >8 METs are associated with 5-year survival of ~95%, which gives physicians the latitude to try less invasive therapies. From the standpoint of prescribing exercise, there is a long tradition of using either the relative heart rate or heart rate reserve, or a normalized approach to exercise capacity (e.g., % heart rate (HR) reserve (% HRR), or % maximal oxygen consumption (% VO_2 max) or maximal METs) [18,19]. For example, in two patients with the same evidence of a disease process (e.g., ST segment depression on the ECG, correlated with chest pain) may be viewed, and treated, very differently depending on their prognosis estimated from exercise capacity.

Table 2. Reasons for exercise testing.

Evaluate Exertional Discomfort
Reduced exercise tolerance
Chest pain
Dyspnea
Claudication
Cerebral symptoms
Reveal Occult Pathology
Change presentation of cardiovascular disease
Define Prognosis
Guide to exercise prescription strategy
Exercise Prescription
Relative percentage concept
Ischemic/arrhythmic threshold

In most cases, maximal exercise is often employed to allow optimization of the diagnostic sensitivity of exercise testing [23] and anchoring of the exercise prescription. However, submaximal testing has been shown to be a valuable alternative when maximal testing is not possible [24] and is certainly less demanding for the patient, may be perceived as safer, and does not require physician involvement. Submaximal exercise outcomes, such as the ventilatory threshold (VT), have become recognized as effective criteria for sustainable exercise capacity [25,26]. Exercise testing in clinical populations is generally thought to be quite safe, with complications requiring medical intervention occurring in ~1% of tests [27] and in healthy individuals/athletes is nearly zero [28]. More recent approaches to using the Rating of Perceived Exertion (RPE) [24,29] and the Talk Test [24,30] to evaluate exercise capacity have appeared and may be just as effective for exercise prescription. For example, an RPE rating of 13-14 or the first time speech comfort is "equivocal" is very close to the VT [24,30]. To the degree that VT may be just as good of an index of sustainable exercise capacity as VO_2 max, such submaximal exercise testing options hold great promise.

3. Exercise Advice vs. Prescription

The value of exercise as a health promoting behavior is large enough that professional societies such as the American College of Sports Medicine, the American Heart Association, and the Centers for Disease Control and Prevention have issued guidelines for public behavior [31,32]. These guidelines, which carry a very favorable benefit–risk ratio, recommend that all adults accumulate at least 150 min of moderate (almost always < VT) intensity exercise, preferably distributed over at least 5 days per week. If one includes ordinary activities as well, this would represent ~10,000 steps per day [12–14] or ~20 METs hours per week [9–11]. It is important to note that these levels of recommendation, which probably approximate 7 h per week, are in excess of the 150 min per week recommended by professional societies [31,32]. The difference may be based on the belief that compliance to recommendations of 150 min per week is likely to be higher than to >400 min per week, and that the public health benefit of more people doing less than idealized exercise is larger than better grounded recommendations which may have lower compliance. These recommendations are not very individually tailored. In many ways, they are comparable to the traditional health recommendations, "an apple a day keeps the doctor away", but have a likely large benefit in terms of health risk, with very minimal likelihood of untoward complications.

However, many people prefer more individually driven exercise prescription. Or in individuals with more fragile clinical conditions, more individually specific advice might be of value. Consistent with the concept of Exercise is Medicine® promoted by the American College of Sports Medicine, there would be some sort of exercise-based evaluation that would allow the generation of an individual exercise prescription. The concept of the American College of Sports Medicine is based on the FITT-VP concept (frequency, intensity, time, type, volume, and progression) [18]. The most difficult of these elements to prescribe is intensity. In the original concept, the intensity of exercise was prescribed based on % of maximal HR (% HRmax), % HRR, % METs, or % MET Reserve [18]. This practice was supported by an abundant data base from randomized trials. However, it requires the presence of a maximal exercise test to anchor the HRmax or max METs, particularly since age-based population estimates of HRmax are known to be individually inadequate [33]. As early as the late 1970s, there were also reports suggesting that exercise prescriptions built on the so-called "relative percent concept" were not very good at creating a homogenous training experience and response [34,35]. Beyond this, it is widely recognized that HRmax achieved during a single incremental bout of exercise (particularly during tests conducted for clinical diagnostics) is unlikely to represent a true HRmax achieved during field testing, or interval training. More recent recommendations have suggested that exercise prescription concepts based on ventilatory/lactate threshold might be superior [25,26,36]. However, determination of "threshold" is technologically demanding, and requires a maximal exercise test. Recent work from our laboratory has suggested that the Talk Test may offer a technologically simple approach to VT estimation [30]. In the Talk Test, it is common to have subjects recite a standard speech passage of ~90 words, and then respond to the question, "can you speak comfortably?". When the subject responds with "yes", they are typically below the intensity of the VT. The first equivocal response, "yes, but", usually occurs at about the intensity of the VT. If the subject responds with a definite "no", the intensity is typically close to the respiratory compensation threshold [30]. Further, work with the RPE has suggested a low-tech way to evaluating either VT or VO_2 max and prescribing exercise that is useful for recommending the intensity of training [25,37,38].

4. Functional Translation

One of the complicating issues when prescribing exercise training, particularly based on responses during submaximal or maximal exercise testing, is that the HR or RPE or Talk Test response at a particular workload during the exercise test "drifts" as exercise is sustained during training. This may be attributable to progressive changes in core temperature, to accumulation of catecholamines, to progressive dehydration, or to other factors related "to fatigue". In other words, a workload that elicits a HR of 130 during exercise testing may have a HR of 145 after 30 min, secondary to cardiovascular drift. This leads to the practical problem of advising patients what to do in the gymnasium based on their exercise test responses. Imagine a person with a resting HR of 50, a maximal HR of 150, and thus a target HR at 70% HRR of 120, with an RPE of 13 and a Talk Test response of "yes, I can talk comfortably". Let us say that this person achieves this HR at 6 min into a standard Bruce treadmill protocol (2.5 mph (4.0 kmh), 12% grade). However, if they go to the gymnasium and begin exercise training at this workload, their HR will quickly be greater than 120, their RPE will be 15 or more, they will not be comfortable talking, and they will have to quit after 15 min or so. Clearly, a prescribed workload will "drift" beyond the scope intended. This highlights the importance of monitoring responses during exercise training via multiple mechanisms (% HRR, RPE, Talk Test). However, sometime the monitoring methods have enough lag that the beginning exerciser gets "behind the curve" and becomes overly fatigued. In an experienced exerciser, this is not a problem. However, in the more vulnerable exerciser, it could provide the substrate for (at least) an unpleasant exercise session, if not an untoward event. If the exercise test responses could be "translated" such that the target workload designed to achieve target values for HR, RPE and Talk Test could be adjusted (down regulated) before the session begins then the response during training might be more optimal.

We have taken this approach with ambulation following a standard treadmill test [38], with cycling after a standard cycle test [38], during arm–leg ergometry [39], during recreational activities [40] for target HR. We have also taken the same approach using the Talk Test as the outcome measure in sedentary individuals [41], well-trained individuals [42], and cardiac patients [30,43,44]. However, the magnitude of the "step down" (down regulation) in workload from exercise testing to exercise training is highly individual and depends on the details of the exercise test protocol. For example, in more rapidly ramped protocols, or in standard clinical protocols (e.g., Bruce treadmill protocols), the lack of near steady state conditions during testing makes the necessity for down-regulating the training session more difficult.

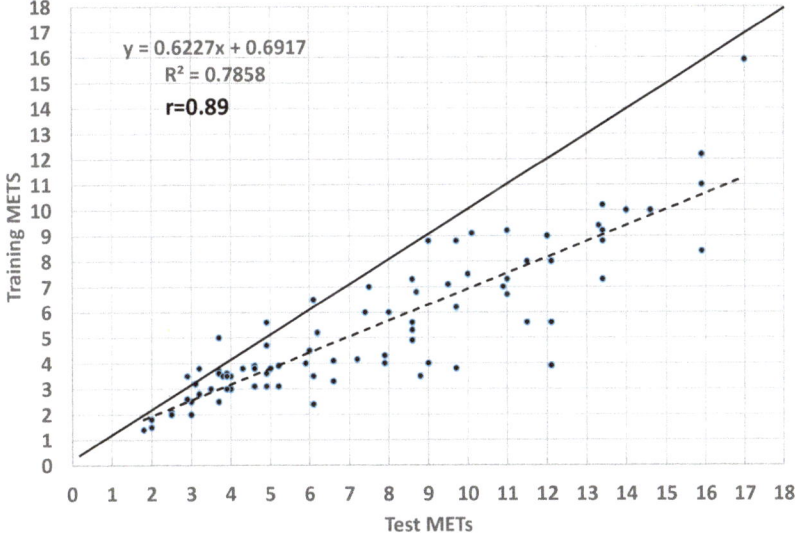

Figure 1. Comparison of exercise intensity (expressed as Metabolic Equivalent Task (METs) during exercise testing and exercise training with the same level of objective exercise intensity (% of Heart Rate Reserve, Rating of Perceived Exertion, Talk Test) based on combined results from several studies [38–44].

In this paper, we have taken the strategy of trying to "generalize" the magnitude of step down, by computing the relative workload, expressed as METs, on the basis of standard metabolic formulas [18] during both exercise testing and training, based on our previously published data [38–44]. We then plotted the METs during the exercise test against the METs during the steady state period (15–30 min) during exercise training, with the same magnitude of homeostatic disturbance in terms of % HRR, Talk Test score, and RPE. The results of this comparison are presented in Figure 1. The translated MET values were well correlated (r = 0.89) and the mean "step down" followed a linear regression, with an average step-down to 71.8% from testing (7.66 ± 4.03 METs) to training (5.50 ± 2.92 METs). This strategy, of course, is primarily designed for near steady state training sessions. In principle it could be extrapolated to interval training, although factors such as the length of the hard and easy segments, as well as the difference between hard and easy segments would have to be considered. Accordingly, the purpose of this study was to develop a 'generalized model' for translating exercise test responses to exercise prescription.

5. Discussion

The main finding of this viewpoint was that it appears possible to generalize previous studies [38–44] intended to "translate" exercise test responses into exercise prescriptions, by expressing the workload as METs. Using this approach, it appears that steady state exercise training at 65–75% of the workload yielding a particular marker of exercise intensity (i.e., % HRR, RPE, Talk Test) during exercise testing will yield comparable responses during exercise training. This problem has not otherwise been widely addressed. However, our results suggest that a larger "stepdown" than the ~10% recommended by Mezzani et al. [24] is necessary. The results are also consistent with the finding of de Koning et al. [45] that VT occurs at about 50% of peak power output (usually ~70% VO_2 max) and that most exercise training, whether for athletes [26] or non-athletes [19], takes place at intensities <VT [20]. Validation of the magnitude of "stepdown" awaits further prospective data.

In the case of already active individuals, the spontaneous choice of the exercise level often yields intensities within commonly recommended guidelines [18]. Indeed, using the Talk Test as a surrogate of exercise intensity, athletic subjects required relatively little adjustment of workload beyond the first moments of the exercise bout [30,42,43]. In other words, in already experienced exercisers, finding the right intensity is relatively simple and rapid. Further, even in minimally trained individuals and cardiac patients, adjustment of the exercise level on the basis of speech comfort yielded appropriate relative MET and % HRR values within a very few minutes of exercise [30,44]. We also know that previously untrained individuals can self-regulate exercise intensity using the RPE scale and achieve an effective training response [37].

In sedentary individuals, unaccustomed heavy exercise can be associated with the "triggering" of myocardial infarction [17]. However, we also know that the incidence of exercise related complications, both in healthy individuals and in cardiac rehabilitation programs, has decreased over time [15], most likely because we are better at regulating exercise intensity during the early weeks of new exercise programs (e.g., avoiding conditions that might promote "triggering" of myocardial infarction). Against the background that many people who have been sedentary for many years and who are beginning an exercise program later in life, and that they may tend to exercise at intensities recalled from earlier in their life. This workload may now be too strenuous and may predispose toward the development of untoward events during training. Thus, rather than prescribing exercise on the basis of % HRR or even RPE, which may take some time to show that the exercise is too strenuous, it would seem to be desirable to have a mechanism for deciding what the appropriate workload should be during the first few days of training, and then fine tuning (e.g., triangulate) this intensity on the basis of conventional monitoring tools (% HRR, RPE, Talk Test).

6. Conclusions

The present results suggest the utility of "translating" exercise test responses into the workload during exercise training that will yield appropriate levels of exercise intensity as defined by % HRR, RPE, or Talk Test. It appears that reducing the workload to 65–75% of that during the exercise test is reasonable and can be done on the basis of METs calculated using standard methods [18]. Particularly in sedentary individuals beginning an exercise program or in patients during rehabilitation, this approach may yield useful estimates of exercise intensity and contribute to both the safety and efficacy of exercise therapy. These data suggest a simple approach to using exercise testing results, which are meaningfully generalized [38–44] from our earlier more specific results. Hopefully, this makes the "functional translation" approach easier to use, although this new approach requires future experimental verification.

Author Contributions: Conceptualization, C.F., J.D.A., D.B.(Daniel Bok), D.B. (Daniel Boullosa), C.C., A.F., J.J.d.K., J.P.P., and J.A.R.-M.; writing-original draft preparation, C.F., G.C., S.J.J., A.L., and K.R.; writing-review and editing, C.F., J.D.A., D.B.(Daniel Bok), D.B. (Daniel Boullosa), G.C., C.C., A.F., S.J.J., J.J.D.K., A.L., J.P.P., K.R., and J.A.R.-M. All authors have read and agreed to the published version of the manuscript.

Funding: This research received no external funding.

Conflicts of Interest: The authors declare no conflict of interest.

References

1. Eaton, S.B.; Konner, M.; Shostak, M. Stone agers in the fast lane: Chronic degenerative diseases in an evolutionary perspective. *Am. J. Med.* **1988**, *84*, 739–749. [CrossRef]
2. Terry, L.L. Surgeon General's Report on Smoking and Tobacco Use. Available online: https://www.cdc.gov/tobacco/data_statistics/sgr/index.htm (accessed on 25 June 2020).
3. Cooper, K.H. *Aerobics*; Bantam Books: New York, NY, USA, 1968.
4. Paffenbarger, R.S.J.; Blair, S.N.; Lee, I.M. A history of physical activity, cardiovascular health and longevity: The scientific contributions of Jeremy N Morris, DSc, DPH, FCCP. *Int. J. Epidemiol.* **2001**, *30*, 1184–1192. [CrossRef] [PubMed]
5. Paffenbarger, R.S.J.; Hale, W.E. Work activity and coronary heart mortality. *N. Engl. J. Med.* **1975**, *292*, 545–550. [CrossRef] [PubMed]
6. Paffenbarger, R.S.J.; Hyde, R.T.; Wing, A.L.; Hsieh, C.C. Physical activity, all-cause mortality and longevity of college alumni. *N. Engl. J. Med.* **1986**, *314*, 605–613. [CrossRef] [PubMed]
7. Blair, S.N.; Kungert, J.B.; Kohl, H.W.; Barlow, C.E.; Macera, C.A.; Paffenbarger Jr, R.S.; Gibbons, L.W. Influences of cardiorespiratory fitness and other precursors of cardiovascular disease and all-cause mortality in men and women. *JAMA* **1996**, *276*, 205–210. [CrossRef]
8. Lee, I.M.; Shiroma, E.J.; Lobelo, F.; Puslza, P.; Blair, S.N.; Katzmarek, P.J. Effect of physical inactivity on major non-communicable diseases worldwide: An analysis of burden of disease and life expectancy. *Lancet* **2012**, *380*, 21–27. [CrossRef]
9. O'Keefe, J.; Lavie, C.J.; Guazzi, M. Potential dangers of extreme endurance exercise: How much is too much? *Prog. Cardiovasc. Dis.* **2015**, *57*, 396–405. [CrossRef]
10. Arem, H.; Moore, S.C.; Patel, A.; Hartge, P.; Berrington de Gonzalez, A.; Visvanathan, K.; Campbell, P.T.; Freedman, M.; Weiderpass, E.; Adami, H.O.; et al. Leisure time physical activity and mortality: A detailed pooled analysis of the dose-response relationship. *JAMA Intern. Med.* **2015**, *175*, 959–967. [CrossRef]
11. Eijsvogels, T.M.; Molossi, S.; Lee, D.C.; Emery, M.S.; Thompson, P.D. Exercise at the extremes: The amount of exercise to reduce cardiovascular events. *J. Am. Coll. Cardiol.* **2016**, *67*, 316–329. [CrossRef]
12. Kraus, W.E.; Janz, K.F.; Powell, K.E.; Campbell, W.W.; Jakicic, J.M.; Troiano, R.P.; Sprow, K.; Torres, A.; Piercy, K.L. Daily step counts for measuring physical activity exposure and its relation to health. *Med. Sci. Sports Exerc.* **2019**, *51*, 1206–1212. [CrossRef]
13. Kraus, W.E.; Powell, K.E.; Haskell, W.L.; Janz, K.F.; Campbell, W.W.; Jakicic, J.M.; Troiano, R.P.; Sprow, K.; Torres, A.; Piercy, K.L. Physical activity and cardiovascular mortality and cardiovascular disease. *Med. Sci. Sports Exerc.* **2019**, *51*, 1270–1281. [CrossRef]
14. Tudor-Locke, C.; Craig, C.L.; Aoyagi, Y.; Bell, R.C.; Croteau, K.A.; De Bourdeaudhuij, I.; Ewald, B.; Gardner, A.W.; Hatano, Y.; Lutes, L.D.; et al. How many steps/day are enough? For older adults and special populations. *Int. J. Behav. Nutr. Phys. Act.* **2011**, *8*, 1–19. [CrossRef] [PubMed]
15. Foster, C.; Porcari, J.P.; Battista, R.A.; Udermann, B.; Wright, G.; Lucia, A. The risk in exercise training. *Am. J. Lifestyle. Med.* **2008**, *2*, 279–284. [CrossRef]

16. Sanchis-Gomar, F.; Pérez, L.M.; Joyner, M.J.; Löllgen, H.; Lucia, A. Endurance exercise and the heart. Friend or foe? *Sports Med.* **2016**, *46*, 459–466. [CrossRef] [PubMed]
17. Thompson, P.D.; Franklin, B.A.; Balady, G.J.; Blair, S.N.; Corrado, D.; Estes, N.A.; Fulton, J.E.; Gordon, N.F.; Haskell, W.L.; Link, M.S.; et al. Exercise and acute cardiovascular events placing the risks into perspective: A scientific statement from the American Heart Association Council on Nutrition, Physical Activity, and Metabolism and the Council on Clinical Cardiology. *Circulation* **2007**, *115*, 2358–2368. [PubMed]
18. ACSM. *ACSM's Guidelines for Exercise Testing and Prescription*, 10th ed.; Wolters Kluwer: Philadelphia, PA, USA, 2017.
19. Foster, C.; Porcari, J.P.; Cress, M. Clinical exercise testing. In *ACSM's Clinical Exercise Physiology*; Thompson, W.R., Ed.; Wolters Kluwer: Baltimore, MD, USA, 2019; pp. 349–364.
20. Meyer, T.; Lucía, A.; Earnest, C.P.; Kindermann, W. A conceptual framework for performance diagnosis and training prescription from submaximal gas exchange parameters-theory and application. *Int. J. Sports Med.* **2005**, *26*, S38–S48. [CrossRef] [PubMed]
21. Myers, J.; Prakash, M.; Froelicher, V.; Do, D.; Partington, S.; Atwood, J.E. Exercise capacity and mortality among men referred for exercise testing. *N. Engl. J. Med.* **2002**, *346*, 793–801. [CrossRef]
22. Mark, D.B.; Shaw, L.; Harrell, F.E.; Hlatky, M.A.; Lee, K.L.; Bengtson, J.R.; McCants, C.B.; Califf, R.M.; Pryor, D.B. Prognostic value of a treadmill exercise score in outpatients with suspected coronary artery disease. *N. Engl. J. Med.* **1991**, *325*, 849–853. [CrossRef]
23. Cumming, G.R. Yield of ischaemic electrocardiograms in relation to exercise intensity in a normal population. *Br. Heart J.* **1972**, *34*, 919–923. [CrossRef]
24. Alajmi, R.A.; Foster, C.; Porcari, J.P.; Radtke, K.; Doberstein, S. Comparison of non-maximal tests for estimating exercise capacity. *Kinesiology* **2020**, *52*, 10–18. [CrossRef]
25. Mezzani, A.; Hamm, L.F.; Jones, A.M.; McBride, P.E.; Moholdt, T.; Stone, J.A.; Urhausen, A.; Williams, M.A. Aerobic exercise intensity assessment and prescription in cardiac rehabilitation: A joint position statement of the European Association for Cardiovascular Prevention and Rehabilitation, the American Association of Cardiovascular and Pulmonary Rehabilitation, and the Canadian Association of Cardiac Rehabilitation. *J. Cardiopulm. Rehabil. Prev.* **2012**, *32*, 327–350. [PubMed]
26. Seiler, S. What is the best practiced for training intensity and duration distribution in endurance athletes? *Int. J. Sports. Physiol. Perform.* **2010**, *5*, 276–291. [CrossRef] [PubMed]
27. Myers, J.; Voodi, L.; Umann, P.A.; Froelicher, V.F. A survey of exercise testing: Methods, utilization, interpretation and safety in the VAHCS. *J. Cardiopulm. Rehabil.* **2000**, *20*, 251–258. [CrossRef]
28. Foster, C. Is there risk in exercise testing of athletes? *Int. J. Sports Physiol. Perform.* **2017**, *12*, 849–850. [CrossRef] [PubMed]
29. Eston, R.; Evans, H.; Faulkner, J.; Lambrick, D.; Al-Rahamneh, G.; Parfitt, G. A perceptually regulated, graded exercise test predicts peak oxygen uptake during treadmill exercise in active and sedentary participants. *Eur. J. Appl. Physiol.* **2012**, *112*, 3459–3468. [CrossRef] [PubMed]
30. Foster, C.; Porcari, J.P.; Doro, K.; Dubiel, J.; Engen, M.; Kolman, D.; Ault, S.; Xiong, S. Exercise prescription when there is no exercise test: The Talk Test. *Kinesiology* **2018**, *50*, 333–348.
31. Pate, R.R.; Pratt, M.; Blair, S.N.; Haskell, W.L.; Macera, C.A.; Bouchard, C.; Buchner, D.; Ettinger, W.; Heath, G.W.; King, A.C. Physical activity and public health. A recommendation from the Centers for Disease Control and Prevention and the American College of Sports Medicine. *JAMA* **1995**, *273*, 402–407. [CrossRef]
32. Haskell, W.L.; Lee, I.M.; Pate, R.R.; Powell, K.E.; Blair, S.N.; Franklin, B.A.; Macera, C.A.; Heath, G.W.; Thompson, P.D.; Bauman, A. Physical activity and public health: Updated recommendation for adults from the American College of Sports Medicine and the American Heart Association. *Med. Sci. Sports Exerc.* **2007**, *39*, 1423–1434. [CrossRef]
33. Robergs, R.A.; Landwehr, R. The surprising history of the "HRmax=220-age" equation. *J. Ex. Phys. Online* **2002**, *5*, 1–10.
34. Katch, V.L.; Weltman, A.; Sady, S.; Freedson, P. Validity of the relative percent concept for equating training intensity. *Eur. J. Appl. Physiol. Occup. Physiol.* **1978**, *39*, 219–227. [CrossRef]
35. Sharhag-Rosenberger, F.; Meyer, T.; Gasler, N.; Faude, O.; Kindermann, W. Exercise at given percentages of VO_2max: Heterogenous metabolic responses between individuals. *J. Sci. Med. Sport* **2010**, *13*, 74–79. [CrossRef] [PubMed]

36. Sylta, Ø.; Tønnessen, E.; Hammarström, D.; Danielsen, J.; Skovereng, K.; Ravn, T.; Rønnestad, B.R.; Sandbakk, Ø.; Seiler, S. The effect of different high-intensity periodization models on endurance adaptations. *Med. Sci. Sports. Exerc.* **2016**, *48*, 2165–2174. [CrossRef] [PubMed]
37. Parfitt, G.; Evans, H.; Eston, R. Perceptually regulated training at RPE13 is pleasant and improves physical health. *Med. Sci. Sports. Exerc.* **2012**, *44*, 1613–1618. [CrossRef] [PubMed]
38. Foster, C.; Lemberger, K.; Thompson, N.N.; Sennett, S.M.; Hare, J.; Pollock, M.L.; Pels, A.E.; Schmidt, D.H. Functional translation of exercise responses from graded exercise testing to exercise training. *Am. Heart J.* **1986**, *112*, 1309–1316. [CrossRef]
39. Foster, C.; Thompson, N.N.; Bales, S. Functional translation of exercise responses using combined arm-leg ergometry. *Cardiology* **1991**, *78*, 150–155. [CrossRef]
40. Foster, C.; Thompson, N.N. Functional translation of exercise test responses to recreational activities. *J. Cardiopulm. Rehabil.* **1991**, *11*, 373–377. [CrossRef]
41. Foster, C.; Porcari, J.P.; Gibson, M.; Wright, G.; Greany, J.; Talati, N.; Recalde, P. Translation of submaximal exercise test responses to exercise prescription using the Talk Test. *J. Strength Cond. Res.* **2009**, *23*, 2425–2429. [CrossRef]
42. Jeans, E.A.; Foster, C.; Porcari, J.P.; Gibson, M.; Doberstein, S. Translation of exercise testing to exercise prescription using the Talk Test. *J. Strength Cond. Res.* **2011**, *25*, 590–596. [CrossRef]
43. Woltmann, M.L.; Foster, C.; Porcari, J.P.; Camic, C.L.; Dodge, C.; Haible, S.; Mikat, R.P. Evidence that the Talk Test can be used to regulated exercise intensity. *J. Strength Cond. Res.* **2015**, *29*, 1248–1254. [CrossRef]
44. Lyon, E.; Menke, M.; Foster, C.; Porcari, J.P.; Gibson, M.; Bubbers, T. Translation of incremental Talk Test responses to steady-state exercise training intensity. *J. Cardiopulm. Rehabil.* **2014**, *34*, 271–275. [CrossRef]
45. De Koning, J.J.; Noorhof, D.A.; Uitslag, T.P.; Gilart, R.E.; Dodge, C.; Foster, C. An approach to estimating gross efficiency during high intensity exercise. *Int. J. Sports Physiol. Perform.* **2013**, *8*, 682–684. [CrossRef] [PubMed]

© 2020 by the authors. Licensee MDPI, Basel, Switzerland. This article is an open access article distributed under the terms and conditions of the Creative Commons Attribution (CC BY) license (http://creativecommons.org/licenses/by/4.0/).

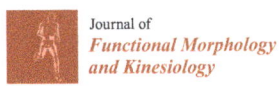

Viewpoint

Perspective of Dose and Response for Individualized Physical Exercise and Training Prescription

Thomas Gronwald [1,*], Alexander Törpel [2], Fabian Herold [3,4] and Henning Budde [5]

1. Faculty of Health Sciences, Department of Performance, Neuroscience, Therapy and Health, MSH Medical School Hamburg, University of Applied Sciences and Medical University, Am Kaiserkai 1, 20457 Hamburg, Germany
2. German Swimming Federation, Korbacher Straße 93, 34132 Kassel, Germany; toerpel@dsv.de
3. Research Group Neuroprotection, German Center for Neurodegenerative Diseases (DZNE), Leipziger Str. 44, 39120 Magdeburg, Germany; fabian.herold@st.ovgu.de
4. Department of Neurology, Medical Faculty, Otto von Guericke University, Leipziger Str. 44, 39120 Magdeburg, Germany
5. Faculty of Human Sciences, MSH Medical School Hamburg, University of Applied Sciences and Medical University, Am Kaiserkai 1, 20457 Hamburg, Germany; henning.budde@medicalschool-hamburg.de
* Correspondence: thomas.gronwald@medicalschool-hamburg.de

Received: 11 June 2020; Accepted: 10 July 2020; Published: 14 July 2020

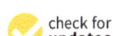

Abstract: Physical interventions are used to increase physical (sports) performance and considered as effective low-cost strategies in the fields of healthcare, disease or injury prevention, and medical treatment. In general, a considerable amount of evidence buttress the application of physical interventions in various fields as it has been demonstrated to contribute to the maintenance and recovery of physical performance, cognitive function, and overall state of health. To implement physical interventions effectively, it is essential to provide an appropriate exercise and training prescription. Exercise and training prescription are key for "dose" specification and for the individualization (personalizing) of physical exercise and training, precisely adjusted and controlled like medication. Since the physiological response to physical interventions is demonstrably individual and dependent on many influencing factors, individualization is an emerging approach aiming to maximize the efficiency of an intervention by accounting for the interindividual heterogeneity. The present brief viewpoint article aims to distinguish and to redefine between the terms dose and response in order to improve the understanding of practitioners, the methodology of study protocols, and to relate future findings to the actual biological (interindividual) variability of acute and chronic responses.

Keywords: dose; acute response; chronic response; internal load; external load; exercise and training prescription; exercise is medicine; personalized medicine

1. Introduction

There is growing evidence that regular physical activity and/or physical exercise (as planned, structured, and purposive forms of physical activity [1,2]) lead to positive effects on physical performance and health in various physiological subsystems (e.g., metabolic, cardiovascular, musculoskeletal, or central nervous system) and the organism as a whole, which emphasizes its use in different fields of application [3,4]. Hence, "physical interventions", which serve as an umbrella term that covers "physical exercise" (as an acute single bout of physical exercise) and "physical training" (as regularly conducted and multiple bouts of physical exercise [2]), are used and have been proven to be an effective low-cost strategy to recover, maintain or increase physical (sports) performance or the overall health status of an individual in different fields of application (e.g., healthcare, disease and injury prevention, medical treatment). To implement physical interventions effectively in physical (sports) performance enhancement, disease prevention, and medical treatments, it is essential to provide an appropriate exercise and training prescription [5,6]. Such a prescription should consider the fundamental principles of exercise and training prescription (e.g., regularity, overload, progression [7]) and should fully specify external load variables (such as exercise and training variables) and internal load variables (see Figure 1). Furthermore, exercise prescription is key for "dose" or "dosage" (regularly provided dose over a specific period of time) specification and for individualization (personalizing) of physical exercise and training, precisely adjusted and controlled like medication [8,9]. In the following, we are using dose as an umbrella term covering dose and dosage.

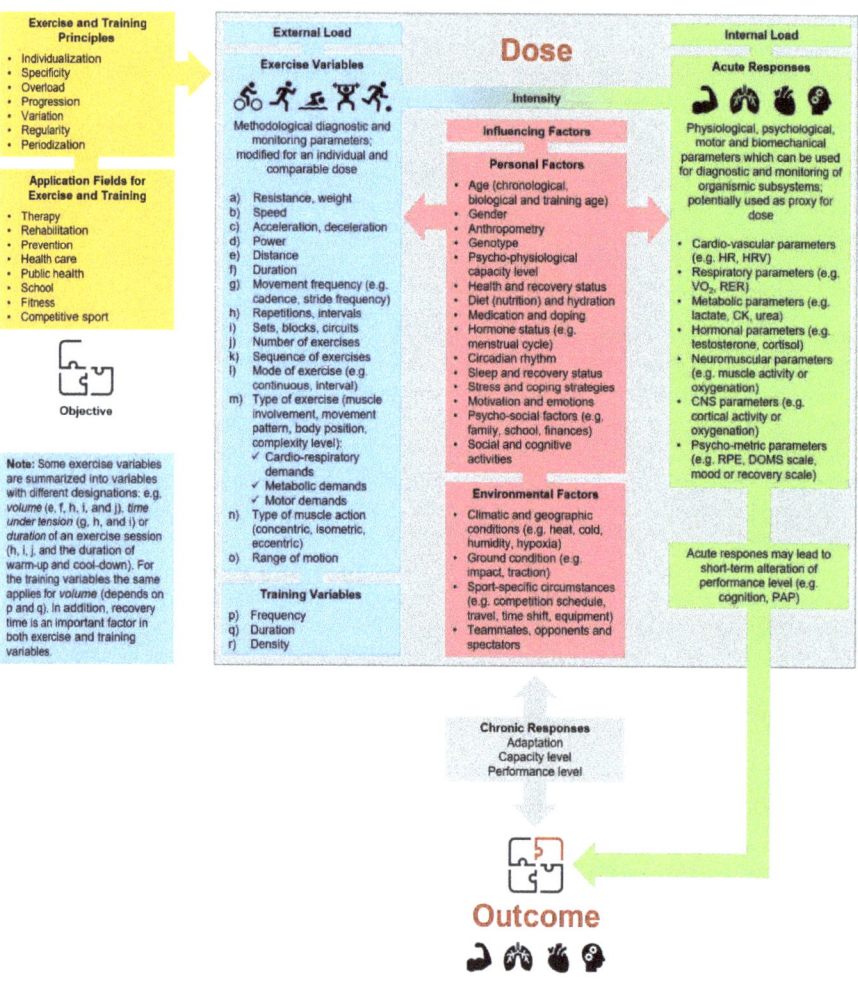

Figure 1. Individual physical exercise and training prescription are based on specific objectives and the respective context in the varying fields of application, as well as principles for the programming and monitoring of physical exercise and training. The dose–outcome relationship depends on a multitude of factors, such as factors of external and internal load and influencing factors. HR: heart rate, HRV: heart rate variability, VO$_2$: oxygen uptake, RER: respiratory exchange ratio, CK: creatine kinase, CNS: central nervous system, RPE: rating of perceived exertion, DOMS: rating of delayed onset muscle soreness, PAP: post-activation potentiation.

Since the physiological response to physical interventions is demonstrably individual and dependent on many influencing factors, individualization is an emerging approach which aims to maximize the efficiency of an intervention by accounting for the interindividual heterogeneity in athletes, healthy populations and patients [5,10–12]. Therefore, it is necessary to evaluate the actual interindividual differences in acute psychophysiological response(s) to the same acute physical exercise and/or adaptations to the same physical training [13–15]. To take interindividual heterogeneity into account, a discussion about the classification of "responder", "non-responder", "adverse responder", or "individuals who did not respond" has been emerged [14,16], but a generally accepted agreement on an appropriate classification approach has yet not been reached [15–17]. However, the extent of the individual physiological response to physical interventions (sensitivity to respond to the given stimuli) need to be referenced relative to a specific outcome in the variable of interest according to the initial objective. The interindividual responsiveness to physical interventions and, in turn, the interindividual heterogeneity in outcomes are caused by several moderators, including non-modifiable factors (e.g., sex or genotype) and modifiable factors (e.g., nutrition, social or cognitive activities, exercise prescription) [13,14,18,19]. Moreover, it is assumed that low-sensitive responsiveness can be best counteracted by modifying the dose of the physical exercise and/or physical training [20,21]. The latter suggests that the dose of physical interventions per se contributes significantly to the observed interindividual heterogeneity of specific outcomes. In a recent systematic review and meta-analysis, Greenham et al. [22] identified biomarkers of physiological responses associated with altered exercise performance following intensified physical training. The majority of the identified biomarkers demonstrated inconsistent findings, due in part to large interindividual response heterogeneity. The authors recommending that future research should strengthens the focus on individual responses rather than group responses and factors that contribute to the interindividual variability in response. In this regard, the term dose of physical interventions has not yet been clearly defined [23]. The present viewpoint article aims to distinguish between the terms dose and response in order to improve the understanding of practitioners and the methodology of study protocols and to relate future findings to the actual biological (interindividual) variability of acute responses and chronic adaptations.

2. Redefining Dose and Response for Individualized Physical Exercise and Training Prescription

An adequate physical exercise and training prescription is a key element in science and practice to characterize the dose of physical interventions. In order to define the dose of a physical intervention, three key components should be considered: (1) external load (defined as the work completed by the individual independent of internal characteristics), (2) influencing factors (all factors that can strengthen or disturb the stimuli of a single bout of exercise and/or training), and (3) internal load (defined as the individual and acute physiological, psychological, motor, and biomechanical responses to the external load and the influencing factors during and/or after the cessation of a single bout of physical exercise) [2,24–30]. Figure 1 gives an overview of the multitude of factors in the subcategories, without claiming to be complete. In this regard, parameters of external load (e.g., running with a speed of 10km/h or swimming with a pace of 65 s per 100 m) or parameters of internal load (e.g., running with 70% of maximum heart rate) can be used to prescribe and control exercise intensity. Here, the internal load has a key role in physical exercise and training prescription as it represents the crucial impetus for acute and/or chronic changes [18,30–34]. Hence, we propose that dose can be operationalized and monitored using a specific indicator (or set of specific indicators) of internal load as proxy. In this regard, it is mandatory to distinguish with respect to the number of exercise sessions between a single bout of physical exercise (i.e., one session leads to an internal load) and repeated bouts of physical exercise defined as training (i.e., several and consecutive sessions during a defined period lead to repeated bouts of internal loads) [1]. Whereas a single bout of physical exercise leads to distinct acute responses shown by a transient reaction of the organism (beneficial, maintaining, or detrimental depending on the stimuli), repeated bouts of physical exercise ultimately converge into distinct chronic responses (beneficial, maintaining, or detrimental depending on the stimuli).

With regard to our definition of dose, and given that internal load as acute response is a part of dose, the term "response" in the frequently used phrase "dose–response" should be specified as "chronic response" (effect on a specific outcome parameter, e.g., mitochondrial volume and density) in the meaning of adaptation as a potential result of several and consecutive sessions of physical exercise. To be even more precise and to broaden the understanding of the dose–response relationship, we recommend redefining the phrase "dose–response" as "dose–outcome", which specifies the link to an acute outcome parameter (in regard to a single bout of physical exercise) or a chronic outcome parameter (in regard to repeated bouts of physical exercise defined as training) according to the respective objective. In this context, dose could be seen as an independent variable or a set of independent variables which we assume to be involved in biological processes in general and in a complex response matrix and signal transduction [35], specifically leading to a distinct "outcome" (dependent variable). However, according to the definitions, internal load as proxy of the dose could be controlled by modifying the external load in consideration of exercise and training principles (e.g., periodization for the planned systematic and structural variation of a training program over time with an adequate ratio of load and recovery periods) and influencing factors such as the actual state of the psychophysiological capacity level (including level of performance).

3. Implications and Areas for Future Research

Valid indicators that represent the most appropriate proxies of dose for prescribing physical interventions are highly specific and more research is needed to identify them (with regard to the context and/or specific acute or chronic responses) [18]. In this regard, current concepts discuss promising internal load parameters (e.g., brain-derived parameters, hormones) to prescribe physical exercise, in addition to traditional measures like heart rate, blood lactate concentration, or rating of perceived exertion [36]. Nevertheless, there is a good, at least theoretical, rationale in support of the individualization of exercise and training prescription by providing a distinct (comparable and standardizable) dose across individuals to elicit the desired psychophysiological responses, which would in turn allow for a better comparison of outcomes across different individuals [2,37,38]. Therefore, existing recommendations endorse the adequate prescription of single exercise sessions and/or training with the specification of parameters of external load and markers of internal load in science and practice [31,32,38,39]. Furthermore, regarding controlled trials of physical interventions and difficulties for blinding participants, it is advisable to include a sham condition in order to avoid potential biases for at least some of a multitude of influencing factors regarding the positive effects of physical activity and physical exercise. A sham intervention should be designed very specifically and should aim to closely replicate virtually all of the elements of a physical exercise condition, regarding variables of physical exercise and physical training (e.g., setting and equipment, socialization, supervision, care, motivation and counselling, outcome expectations, modality and type of exercise, volume, duration, movement frequency, training frequency and density, e.g., [18,40,41]), with the exception of important (hypothesized) prescriptive elements leading to targeted outcomes (e.g., exercise intensity, progression over time). Promising methodological approaches already exist for this purpose [42]. The importance of controlling for social support when designing interventions, which points out the need for adequate sham intervention, has also been highlighted by different authors [43,44]. This approach will further ensure high quality standards for the evaluation of exercise and training prescription and the dose effects of physical interventions.

4. Conclusions

In essence, this brief opinion provides a new and clearer definition of the terms dose and response in the context of exercise and training prescription. We propose that the dose of physical exercise and/or physical training should be operationalized by a specific marker (or specific markers) of internal load. Modifying the exercise prescription by carefully adjusting the external load, a comparable dose can be achieved across individuals, discovering the "real" interindividual heterogeneity regarding acute and chronic responses to physical interventions. We strongly encourage researcher to investigate whether exercise and training prescription that induces a comparable dose may reduce the interindividual heterogeneity considering specific (targeted) outcome variables [45].

Author Contributions: Substantial contributions to the conception and design of the work: T.G., A.T., and F.H. First draft of the work: T.G. Revisiting it critically for important intellectual content: T.G., A.T., F.H., and H.B. All authors have read and approved the final version of the manuscript and agree to the order of presentation of the authors.

Funding: This research received no external funding.

Acknowledgments: We want to acknowledge the enriching discussion with our students of sports sciences (Medical School Hamburg, Otto von Guericke University Magdeburg) and colleagues that helped us to push forward the idea to develop this viewpoint article and to refine our thoughts with regard to the "dose–response" relationship in physical exercise and training prescription.

Conflicts of Interest: The authors declare no conflict of interest.

References

1. Budde, H.; Schwarz, R.; Velasques, B.; Ribeiro, P.; Holzweg, M.; Machado, S.; Brazaitis, M.; Staack, F.; Wegner, M. The need for differentiating between exercise, physical activity, and training. *Autoimmun. Rev.* **2016**, *15*, 110–111. [CrossRef]
2. Gronwald, T.; Budde, H. Commentary: Physical exercise as personalized medicine for dementia prevention? *Front. Physiol.* **2019**, *10*, 1358. [CrossRef]
3. Pedersen, B.K.; Saltin, B. Exercise as medicine—Evidence for prescribing exercise as therapy in 26 different chronic diseases. *Scand. J. Med. Sci. Sports* **2015**, *25*, 1–72. [CrossRef] [PubMed]
4. Luan, X.; Tian, X.; Zhang, H.; Huang, R.; Li, N.; Chen, P.; Wang, R. Exercise as a prescription for patients with various diseases. *J. Sport Health Sci.* **2019**, *8*, 422–441. [CrossRef] [PubMed]
5. Buford, T.W.; Roberts, M.D.; Church, T.S. Toward exercise as personalized medicine. *Sports Med.* **2013**, *43*, 157–165. [CrossRef] [PubMed]
6. Zubin Maslov, P.; Schulman, A.; Lavie, C.J.; Narula, J. Personalized exercise dose prescription. *Eur. Heart J.* **2018**, *39*, 2346–2355. [CrossRef]
7. Kasper, K. Sports Training Principles. *Curr. Sports Med. Rep.* **2019**, *18*, 95–96. [CrossRef]
8. Wasfy, M.M.; Baggish, A.L. Exercise dose in clinical practice. *Circulation* **2016**, *133*, 2297–2313. [CrossRef]
9. Pontifex, M.B.; McGowan, A.L.; Chandler, M.C.; Gwizdala, K.L.; Parks, A.C.; Fenn, K.; Kamijo, K. A primer on investigating the after effects of acute bouts of physical activity on cognition. *Psychol. Sport Exerc.* **2018**, *40*, 1–22. [CrossRef]
10. Lightfoot, J.T. Commentary on viewpoint: Perspective on the future use of genomics in exercise prescription. *J. Appl. Physiol.* **2008**, *104*, 1249. [CrossRef]
11. Barha, C.K.; Galea, L.A.; Nagamatsu, L.S.; Erickson, K.I.; Liu-Ambrose, T. Personalising exercise recommendations for brain health: Considerations and future directions. *Br. J. Sports Med.* **2017**, *51*, 636–639. [CrossRef] [PubMed]
12. Bogataj, Š.; Pajek, M.; Pajek, J.; Buturović Ponikvar, J.; Paravlic, A.H. Exercise-Based Interventions in Hemodialysis Patients: A Systematic Review with a Meta-Analysis of Randomized Controlled Trials. *J. Clin. Med.* **2020**, *9*, 43. [CrossRef] [PubMed]
13. Sparks, L.M. Exercise training response heterogeneity: Physiological and molecular insights. *Diabetologia* **2017**, *60*, 2329–2336. [CrossRef]
14. Pickering, C.; Kiely, J. Do Non-Responders to Exercise Exist-and If So, What Should We Do About Them? *Sports Med.* **2019**, *49*, 1–7. [CrossRef] [PubMed]
15. Ross, R.; Goodpaster, B.H.; Koch, L.G.; Sarzynski, M.A.; Kohrt, W.M.; Johannsen, N.M.; Skinner, J.S.; Castro, A.; Irving, B.A.; Noland, R.C.; et al. Precision exercise medicine: Understanding exercise response variability. *Br. J. Sports Med.* **2019**, *53*, 1141–1153. [CrossRef]
16. Atkinson, G.; Williamson, P.; Batterham, A.M. Issues in the determination of 'responders' and 'non-responders' in physiological research. *Exp. Physiol.* **2019**, *104*, 1215–1225. [CrossRef] [PubMed]
17. Voisin, S.; Jacques, M.; Lucia, A.; Bishop, D.J.; Eynon, N. Statistical considerations for exercise protocols aimed at measuring trainability. *Exerc. Sports Sci. Rev.* **2019**, *47*, 37–45. [CrossRef] [PubMed]

18. Herold, F.; Müller, P.; Gronwald, T.; Müller, N.G. Dose-response matters!—A perspective on the exercise prescription in exercise-cognition research. *Front. Psychol.* **2019**, *10*, 2338. [CrossRef]
19. Mann, T.N.; Lamberts, R.P.; Lambert, M.I. High responders and low responders: Factors associated with individual variation in response to standardized training. *Sports Med.* **2014**, *44*, 1113–1124. [CrossRef]
20. Ross, R.; de Lannoy, L.; Stotz, P.J. Separate Effects of Intensity and Amount of Exercise on Interindividual Cardiorespiratory Fitness Response. *Mayo Clin. Proc.* **2015**, *90*, 1506–1514. [CrossRef]
21. Montero, D.; Lundby, C. Refuting the myth of non-response to exercise training: 'non-responders' do respond to higher dose of training. *J. Physiol.* **2017**, *595*, 3377–3387. [CrossRef] [PubMed]
22. Greenham, G.; Buckley, J.D.; Garrett, J.; Eston, R.; Norton, K. Biomarkers of physiological responses to periods of intensified, non-resistance-based exercise training in well-trained male athletes: A systematic review and meta-analysis. *Sports Med.* **2018**, *48*, 2517–2548. [CrossRef]
23. Voils, C.I.; Chang, Y.; Crandell, J.; Leeman, J.; Sandelowski, M.; Maciejewski, M.L. Informing the dosing of interventions in randomized trials. *Contemp. Clin. Trials* **2012**, *33*, 1225–1230. [CrossRef]
24. Halson, S.L. Monitoring training load to understand fatigue in athletes. *Sports Med.* **2014**, *44*, 139–147. [CrossRef] [PubMed]
25. Soligard, T.; Schwellnus, M.; Alonso, J.-M.; Bahr, R.; Clarsen, B.; Dijkstra, H.P.; Gabbett, T.; Gleeson, M.; Hägglund, M.; Hutchinson, M.R.; et al. How much is too much? (Part 1) International Olympic Committee consensus statement on load in sport and risk of injury. *Br. J. Sports Med.* **2016**, *50*, 1030–1041. [CrossRef]
26. Burgess, D.J. The Research Doesn't Always Apply: Practical Solutions to Evidence-Based Training-Load Monitoring in Elite Team Sports. *Int. J. Sports Physiol. Perf.* **2017**, *12*, S2136–S2141. [CrossRef] [PubMed]
27. Bourdon, P.C.; Cardinale, M.; Murray, A.; Gastin, P.; Kellmann, M.; Varley, M.C.; Gabbett, T.J.; Coutts, A.J.; Burgess, D.J.; Gregson, W.; et al. Monitoring Athlete Training Loads: Consensus Statement. *Int. J. Sports Physiol. Perf.* **2017**, *12*, S161–S170. [CrossRef] [PubMed]
28. Vanrenterghem, J.; Nedergaard, N.J.; Robinson, M.A.; Drust, B. Training Load Monitoring in Team Sports: A Novel Framework Separating Physiological and Biomechanical Load-Adaptation Pathways. *Sports Med.* **2017**, *47*, 2135–2142. [CrossRef]
29. McLaren, S.J.; Macpherson, T.W.; Coutts, A.J.; Hurst, C.; Spears, I.R.; Weston, M. The Relationships Between Internal and External Measures of Training Load and Intensity in Team Sports: A Meta-Analysis. *Sports Med.* **2018**, *48*, 641–658. [CrossRef]
30. Impellizzeri, F.M.; Marcora, S.M.; Coutts, A.J. Internal and External Training Load: 15 Years On. *Int. J. Sports Physiol. Perf.* **2019**, *14*, 270–273. [CrossRef]
31. Banister, E.W.; Calvert, T.W.; Savage, M.V.; Bach, T. A system model of training for athletic performance. *Aust. J. Sports Med.* **1975**, *7*, 57–61.
32. Foster, C.; Florhaug, J.A.; Franklin, J.; Gottschall, L.; Hrovatin, L.A.; Parker, S.; Doleshal, P.; Dodge, C. A new approach to monitoring exercise training. *J. Strength Cond. Res.* **2001**, *15*, 109–115.
33. Borresen, J.; Lambert, M.I. The quantification of training load, the training response and the effect on performance. *Sports Med.* **2009**, *39*, 779–795. [CrossRef] [PubMed]
34. Foster, C.; Rodriguez-Marroyo, J.A.; de Koning, J.J. Monitoring training loads: The past, the present, and the future. *Int. J. Sports Physiol. Perform.* **2017**, *12*, S22–S28. [CrossRef] [PubMed]
35. Toigo, M.; Boutellier, U. New fundamental resistance exercise determinants of molecular and cellular muscle adaptations. *Eur. J. Appl. Physiol.* **2006**, *97*, 643–663. [CrossRef] [PubMed]
36. Herold, F.; Gronwald, T.; Scholkmann, F.; Zohdi, H.; Wyser, D.; Müller, N.G.; Hamacher, D. New Directions in Exercise Prescription: Is There a Role for Brain-Derived Parameters Obtained by Functional Near-Infrared Spectroscopy? *Brain Sci.* **2020**, *10*, 342. [CrossRef]
37. Gronwald, T.; Velasques, B.; Ribeiro, P.; Machado, S.; Murillo-Rodriguez, E.; Ludyga, S.; Yamamoto, T.; Budde, H. Increasing exercise's effect on mental health: Exercise intensity does matter! *PNAS* **2018**, *115*, E11890–E11891. [CrossRef]
38. Gronwald, T.; de Bem Alves, A.C.; Murillo-Rodriguez, E.; Latini, A.; Schuette, J.; Budde, H. Standardization of exercise intensity and consideration of a dose-response is essential. Commentary on "Exercise-linked FNDC5/irisin rescues synaptic plasticity and memory defects in Alzheimer's models", by Lourenco et al. published 2019 in Nature Medicine. *J. Sport Health Sci.* **2019**, *8*, 353–354. [CrossRef]
39. Impellizzeri, F.M.; Rampinini, E.; Coutts, A.J.; Sassi, A.; Marcora, S.M. Use of RPE-based training load in soccer. *Med. Sci. Sports Exerc.* **2004**, *36*, 1042–1047. [CrossRef]

40. Bogataj, Š.; Pajek, J.; Ponikvar, J.B.; Hadžić, V.; Pajek, M. Kinesiologist-guided functional exercise in addition to intradialytic cycling program in end-stage kidney disease patients: A randomised controlled trial. *Sci. Rep.* **2020**, *10*, 1–10. [CrossRef]
41. Bogataj, Š.; Pajek, M.; Buturović Ponikvar, J.; Pajek, J. Outcome Expectations for Exercise and Decisional Balance Questionnaires Predict Adherence and Efficacy of Exercise Programs in Dialysis Patients. *Int. J. Envorin. Res. Public Health* **2020**, *17*, 3175.
42. Lange, A.K.; Vanwanseele, B.; Foroughi, N.; Baker, M.K.; Shnier, R.; Smith, R.M.; Singh, M.A.F. Resistive Exercise for Arthritic Cartilage Health (REACH): A randomized double-blind, sham-exercise controlled trial. *BMC Geriatrics* **2009**, *9*, 1. [CrossRef] [PubMed]
43. Budde, H.; Akko, D.P.; Ainamani, H.E.; Murillo-Rodríguez, E.; Weierstall, R. The impact of an exercise training intervention on cortisol levels and post-traumatic stress disorder in juveniles from an Ugandan refugee settlement: Study protocol for a randomized control trial. *Trials* **2018**, *19*, 364. [CrossRef] [PubMed]
44. Wegner, M.; Amatriain-Fernández, S.; Kaulitzky, A.; Murillo-Rodriguez, E.; Machado, S.; Budde, H. Systematic review of meta-analyses: Exercise effects on depression in children and adolescents. *Front. Psych.* **2020**, *11*, 81. [CrossRef] [PubMed]
45. Herold, F.; Törpel, A.; Hamacher, D.; Budde, H.; Gronwald, T. A Discussion on Different Approaches for Prescribing Physical Interventions—Four Roads Lead to Rome, but Which One Should We Choose? *J. Pers. Med.* **2020**, *10*, 55. [CrossRef]

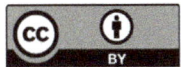

© 2020 by the authors. Licensee MDPI, Basel, Switzerland. This article is an open access article distributed under the terms and conditions of the Creative Commons Attribution (CC BY) license (http://creativecommons.org/licenses/by/4.0/).

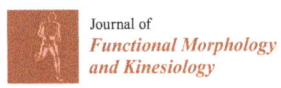

Journal of
Functional Morphology and Kinesiology

Article

Effects of a Supervised Nordic Walking Program on Obese Adults with and without Type 2 Diabetes: The C.U.R.I.A.Mo. Centre Experience

Roberto Pippi [1,†], Andrea Di Blasio [2,†], Cristina Aiello [1], Carmine Fanelli [1], Valentina Bullo [3], Stefano Gobbo [3,*], Lucia Cugusi [4,‡] and Marco Bergamin [3,‡]

1. Healthy Lifestyle Institute, C.U.R.I.A.Mo (Centro Universitario Ricerca Interdipartimentale Attività Motoria), University of Perugia, Via G. Bambagioni, 19 06126 Perugia, Italy; roberto.pippi@unipg.it (R.P.); cristina.aiello@hotmail.com (C.A.); carmine.fanelli@unipg.it (C.F.)
2. Department of Medicine and Aging Sciences, 'G. d'Annunzio' University of Chieti-Pescara, 66100 Chieti Scalo, Italy; andiblasio@gmail.com
3. Department of Medicine, Sport and Exercise Medicine Division, University of Padova, Via Giustiniani 2, 35128 Padova, Italy; valentina.bullo@unipd.it (V.B.); marco.bergamin@unipd.it (M.B.)
4. Department of Biomedical Sciences, University of Sassari, 07100 Sassari, Italy; lucia.cugusi@uniss.it
* Correspondence: stefano.gobbo@unipd.it
† These authors equally contributed to this manuscript.
‡ These authors equally contributed to this manuscript.

Received: 28 May 2020; Accepted: 6 August 2020; Published: 7 August 2020

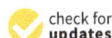

Abstract: Exercise is a convenient non-medical intervention, commonly recommended in metabolic syndrome and type 2 diabetes (DM2) managements. Aerobic exercise and aerobic circuit training have been shown to be able to reduce the risk of developing DM2-related complications. Growing literature proves the usefulness of Nordic walking as exercise therapy in different disease populations, therefore it has a conceivable use in DM2 management. Aims of this study were to analyze and report the effects of two different supervised exercises (gym-based exercise and Nordic walking) on anthropometric profile, blood pressure values, blood chemistry and fitness variables in obese individuals with and without DM2. In this study, 108 obese adults (aged 45–65 years), with or without DM2, were recruited and allocated into one of four subgroups: (1) Gym-based exercise program ($n = 49$) or (2) Nordic walking program ($n = 37$) for obese adults; (3) Gym-based exercise program ($n = 10$) or (4) Nordic walking program ($n = 12$) for obese adults with DM2. In all exercise subgroups, statistically significant improvements in body weight, body mass index, fat mass index, muscular flexibility and maximal oxygen uptake (VO_2 max) were observed. Moreover, a higher percentage of adherence to the gym-based program compared to Nordic walking was recorded. Our findings showed that, notwithstanding the lower adherence, a supervised Nordic walk is effective as a conventional gym-based program to improve body weight control, body composition parameters, muscular flexibility and VO_2 max levels in obese adults with and without type 2 diabetes.

Keywords: Nordic walking; obesity; type 2 diabetes; cardiometabolic fitness

1. Introduction

Physical inactivity is one of the most common risk factors that increase the risk of developing relevant non-communicable diseases (e.g., type 2 diabetes, DM2) and their related risk of mortality [1]. In 2019, the International Diabetes Federation (IDF) estimated that approximately 463 million people have diabetes (type 1 and 2, diagnosed and undiagnosed) worldwide [2]. To counteract and contain this phenomenon, worldwide actions aimed to promote specific health prevention interventions.

These interventions aim to reduce cardiometabolic risk factors, combining a balanced diet with an adequate level of weekly physical activity (PA), and drugs consumption where necessary.

Exercise is an effective non-medical intervention for the management of metabolic syndrome and DM2 [3,4]. In fact, aerobic exercise is the most studied type of exercise and most prescribed in people with common non-communicable chronic diseases, and it has shown to elicit beneficial effects in metabolic, Hb1Ac, body weight and insulin resistance control, also improving fat distribution and microcirculatory function [5,6], with a major effect achieved when combined with resistance training [7,8]. Moreover, aerobic exercise is able to lower the risk of DM2-related complications, such as diabetic nephropathy, retinopathy and neuropathy [9].

Walking is one of the most common physical activities, rarely associated with physical injuries due to its executive characteristics [10]. It can be performed in different environments with no need for particular equipment, overcoming some common barriers such as lack of time, low fitness level, and shortage of money. Walking is able to increase insulin sensitivity and reduces many cardiovascular risk factors, such as hypertension, dyslipidemia and fat mass accumulation [11–13].

Therefore, studying the effects of a particular type of walking practice, such as Nordic walking (NW), could be useful and could help to set an exercise prescription for NW practitioners. NW is an easy-to-learn activity that can be practiced anywhere and only requires the practitioner to be equipped with specific poles. NW involves upper and lower limbs simultaneously, with an increase of approximately 23% in energy expenditure compared to common walking activity [14,15], potentially ensuring major positive physiological effects linked with the prolonged and contemporaneous use of big muscle masses. Several studies showed the beneficial effects of NW in different disease populations [15–19], but only a few studies have investigated the cardiometabolic effects of NW in individuals with obesity and DM2 [20–23]. So, the aims of our study were to analyze and report the cardiometabolic effects following a multidisciplinary intervention performed at the Centro Universitario Ricerca Interdipartimentale Attività Motoria (C.U.R.I.A.Mo.) center, which included two different forms of supervised exercise programs (NW outdoor and exercise indoor) for individuals with obesity and DM2. The cardiometabolic effects of NW activity were compared with those aroused from a conventional exercise-based intervention performed indoor (gym-based exercise, GYM), which combined aerobic and resistance exercises.

2. Materials and Methods

2.1. Participants

From 2010 to 2014, a total sample of 108 obese adults (73 women and 35 men) with and without DM2 (mean age of 56.44 ± 5.94 years) were recruited at the C.U.R.I.A.Mo. center to follow an intensive and multidisciplinary intervention protocol (Figure 1), comprising Nordic walking (NW) and a gym-based exercise program (GYM).

Inclusion criteria were: age between 45 and 65 years and a body mass index (BMI) ≥ 30 kg/m². The exclusion criteria were: presence of musculoskeletal disorders or other clinical conditions that could seriously reduce life expectancy or their ability to participate in the study. Women were 45–65 years old (mean age = 56.37), but no data about menopause were collected, and the statistical analyses conducted, revealed no age effects on the considered variables both at T0 and T1.

In accordance with the subjects' clinical conditions, which were evaluated during the first medical examination (obese individuals with or without DM2), and the different forms of exercise programs proposed (NW or GYM), participants were allocated into 1 of the 4 subgroups:

1. Gym-based exercise program for obese individuals (OB-GYM; $n = 49$);
2. NW program for obese individuals (OB-NW; $n = 37$);
3. Gym-based exercise program for obese individuals with DM2 (DM2-GYM; $n = 10$);
4. NW program for obese individuals with DM2 (DM2-NW; $n = 12$).

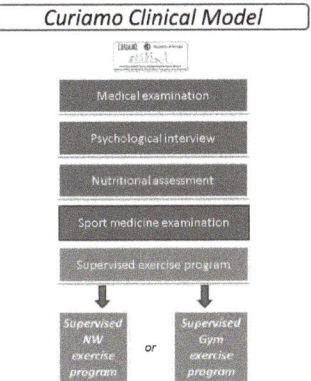

Figure 1. The "Centro Universitario Ricerca Interdipartimentale Attività Motoria" clinical model (De Feo et al., JEI 2011 [24]).

The baseline characteristics of participants are shown in Table 1.

2.2. Study Design

The C.U.R.I.A.Mo. clinical model, previously described by De Feo [24], provides the participation of master-trained specialists, who work following a multidisciplinary method. The C.U.R.I.A.Mo. project has been registered in the Australian New Zealand Clinical Trials Registry (a Primary Registry in the WHO registry network), with the number: ACTRN12611000255987.

All the participants gave their written informed consent to participate in the study, and prior to starting any kind of assessments, were asked to fill out a questionnaire regarding the possible presence of musculoskeletal disorders, which could influence our choice when assigning the subjects to either the GYM or NW program. Using a quasi-experimental study design, individuals were assessed before (T0) and at the end of each exercise intervention (T1).

2.3. The C.U.R.I.A.Mo. Clinical Model

All the participants have been assessed through the C.U.R.I.A.Mo. evaluation model composed by four clinical steps.

1. A medical examination was managed by the endocrinologist to exclude the presence of clinical conditions that could contraindicate the exercise interventions. During the visit, the C.U.R.I.A.Mo. clinical model was explained to participants, and the blood tests were prescribed according to national standards of care [25].
2. A psychological interview to increase the subjects' lifestyle change and to assess their psychological status.
3. A nutritional evaluation to assess the nutritional habits of the participants in order to increase their awareness of a balanced daily diet based on the Mediterranean dietary principles. The C.U.R.I.A.Mo. model provides two individual counseling sessions (before and after the interventions). Nutritional counseling aims to reduce saturated and trans-unsaturated fatty acids to under 10% of the total daily energy, promoting the consumption of fish, vegetables, legumes, fruit and whole grain cereals, to reduce calorie intake. Participants were also invited to attend educational classes focused on healthy diets and good physical activity habits.
4. A complete medical examination was performed by a physician focused on assessing the individual aerobic capacity and muscle strength, and to exclude any potential contraindications to exercise. These outcomes were also used to increase the participants' awareness of their individual physical status.

Table 1. Anthropometric, blood pressure, blood chemistry, and fitness parameters at baseline. **Baseline values:** Mean values of anthropometric, blood pressure and blood chemistry parameters in the entire sample and in the 4 subgroups. Data are presented as means ± SDs. Statistical significance was set for p values ≤ 0.05.

Outcomes	Total Sample $n = 108$ (F = 73; M = 35)	OB-GYM $n = 49$ (F = 33; M = 16)	OB-NW $n = 37$ (F = 30; M = 7)	DM2-GYM $n = 10$ (F = 4; M = 6)	DM2-NW $n = 12$ (F = 6; M = 6)	F	p Values
Age	56.44 ± 5.94	55.29 ± 5.67	56.62 ± 5.8	59.6 ± 6.5	58 ± 6.35	1.89	0.14
Body weight (kg)	100.75 ± 15.4	101.07 ± 16.71	98.50 ± 14.87	104.51 ± 14.38	103.23 ± 12.58	0.57	0.64
BMI (kg/m^2)	36.47 ± 5.11	36.6 ± 4.99	36.37 ± 5.85	35.48 ± 4.32	37.07 ± 4.07	0.19	0.90
FM index (kg of fat mass/m^2)	15.27 ± 4.24	15.22 ± 3.91	15.74 ± 4.64	13.62 ± 4.16	15.46 ± 4.6	0.65	0.58
FFM index (kg of fat free mass/m^2)	19.87 ± 2.27	20.05 ± 2.23	19.15 ± 1.99	20.77 ± 2.91	20.49 ± 2.36	2.17	0.08
Waist circumference (cm)	115.93 ± 10.52	114.88 ± 11.26	115.5 ± 9.83	118.5 ± 9.88	119.25 ± 10.22	0.77	0.51
Waist–Height Ratio	0.7 ± 0.06	0.69 ± 0.07	0.7 ± 0.07	0.69 ± 0.06	0.72 ± 0.07	0.49	0.69
SBP (mmHg)	135 ± 13.08	134.69 ± 10.43	135 ± 12.95	137 ± 16.02	134.55 ± 21.27	0.09	0.97
DBP (mmHg)	82.52 ± 8.94	83.64 ± 7.83	80.86 ± 9.66	85 ± 7.07	80.46 ± 12.14	1.13	0.34
Fasting blood glucose (mg/dL)	105.13 ± 30.83	95 ± 12.64	94.62 ± 11.66	149 ± 58.25	138.83 ± 35.45	24.58	<0.01
HbA1c (%)	6.04 ± 0.99	5.71 ± 0.52	5.76 ± 0.41	7.17 ± 1.91	7 ± 1.07	15.17	<0.01
Total cholesterol (mg/dL)	210.76 ± 36.78	218.06 ± 35.26	207.91 ± 35.67	201.9 ± 41.52	196.67 ± 39.9	1.52	0.22
HDL cholesterol (mg/dL)	49.65 ± 11.48	49.83 ± 9.99	53.06 ± 13.86	43.1 ± 8.89	44.75 ± 8.07	2.98	0.04
Triglycerides (mg/dL)	151.81 ± 82.19	142.49 ± 66.51	130.67 ± 46.22	253.9 ± 169.79	162.92 ± 53.07	7.28	<0.01
Vertical bending (cm)	−9.67 ± 9.34	−9.89 ± 9.31	−6 ± 2	−12 ± 10.61	−8.6 ± 13.33	0.51	0.68
Horizontal bending (cm)	24.89 ± 9.72	24.26 ± 8.83	33.33 ± 7.06	21 ± 9.53	27 ± 15.68	2.26	0.09
VO$_2$ max (mL/kg/min)	13.98 ± 9.25	14.40 ± 8.77	11.88 ± 12.85	14.77 ± 12	11.6 ± 2.85	0.16	0.92

Abbreviations: F: females; M: males; OB-GYM: individuals with obesity participating at gym-based exercise program; OB-NW: individuals with obesity participating in the Nordic walking exercise program; DM2-GYM: obese individuals with DM2 participating in the gym-based exercise program; DM2-NW: obese individuals with DM2 participating in the Nordic walking program; BMI: body mass index; FM: fat mass; FFM: fat-free mass; SBP: systolic blood pressure; DBP: diastolic blood pressure; HbA1c: glycosylated hemoglobin; HDL: high-density lipoprotein; VO$_2$ max: maximal oxygen.

2.4. Exercise Interventions

The two forms of supervised exercise programs (NW and GYM) were planned in accordance with the main international guidelines on exercise prescriptions (American College of Sport Medicine, ACSM) and other previous studies [7,26–28]. Both indoor (GYM) and outdoor (NW) programs were supervised by a specialist sports science graduate. Blood pressure and blood glucose values were recorded at the beginning and at the end of each training session. All the participants were constantly monitored through a heart rate (HR) monitor to ensure that the training program was performed according to the target intensity suggested by ACSM [26]. Furthermore, adherence to each exercise program was recorded and calculated. Specific reports about the two interventions are presented in Table 2.

Table 2. Exercises for both Nordic walking (NW) program and gym-based exercise program (GYM).

Phase	Exercise	Duration	Sets	Repetitions	Intensity
Nordic Walking					
Warm up		10 min			
Main part	Nordic walking	60–65 min			40 to 60% HRR
Cool down	Stretching	15 min			
GYM Program					
Warm up	Treadmill, or walking, or cycling	10 min			
Main part	Treadmill	12 min			40 to 60% HRR
	Leg press		2	20	55 to 70% 1-RM
	Cycle ergometer	4 min			40 to 60% HRR
	Lat machine		2	20	55 to 70% 1-RM
	Arm ergometer	4 min			40 to 60% HRR
	Chest press		2	20	55 to 70% 1-RM
	Cardio	4 min			40 to 60% HRR
	Abdominal		3	10–15	55 to 70% 1-RM
	Cardio	4 min			40 to 60% HRR
	Leg extension		2	20	55 to 70% 1-RM
Cool down	Treadmill, or walking, or cycling Stretching	15 min			

Abbreviations: HRR: heart rate reserve; 1RM: 1-repetition maximum.

2.4.1. Nordic Walking Program

The Nordic walking program was performed on a 750 m-long circular path that was located in the natural park area of the Bambagioni Sporting Centre at the University of Perugia. Exercise sessions were performed 2 times per week and lasted 90 min (10 min of warm up, 60–65 min of NW, and 15 min of cool down). The training intensity was gradually increased, starting from 40% up to 60% of the HR reserve (calculated using the Karvonen formula [29]), through gradual steps of increment. Before the training program, 2 weeks were dedicated to a familiarization with the NW technique.

2.4.2. GYM Program

The gym-based exercise program was planned as a combined circuit training protocol, performed 2 times per week, and lasted 90 min. Before and after the circuit training protocol, 10 min of warm up and 15 min of cool down aerobic exercise (walking, or treadmill, or cycling) were performed.

The main part of the sessions consisted of a set of exercises involving the large muscle groups of the lower and upper limbs; the circuit training mixed aerobic and strength exercise, alternating six aerobic exercises (e.g., cycling and walking) and five strength exercise stations (e.g., leg press, abdominal exercises, pectoral exercises performed with isotonic machines and free weights). Aerobic exercise intensity was monitored and gradually increased, as in the NW protocol. In addition, strength training intensity increased gradually, starting from 55% of one repetition maximum (1-RM) and, in time, up to 70%. Brzycki equation was used to predict the 1-RM estimated value (1-RM = 100 × (load repetition, or workload value of repetition performance, expressed in kg)/(102.78 − 2.78 * number of repetitions performed)) [30].

2.5. Specific Functional and Clinical Assessments

Before starting and at the end of the two exercise interventions all participants underwent a clinical and functional assessment. Anthropometric parameters included waist circumference (WC), height, body weight (BW), body mass index (BMI), and waist–height ratio (WHR) evaluated using standard techniques [31–33]. Body composition (fat mass and fat-free mass indexes) was also evaluated through the use of the Tanita body composition analyzer BC-420MA (Tokyo, Japan) [34]. Systolic and diastolic blood pressure (BP) values were measured through a UM-101 mercury-free sphygmomanometer (A&D Medical, Tokyo, Japan) during the first ambulatory visit. Blood chemistry variables, such as fasting blood glucose, glycated hemoglobin (HbA1c), total cholesterol, high-density lipoprotein (HDL) cholesterol and triglycerides were collected in the laboratory analyses report. Fitness variables, such as aerobic fitness (maximal oxygen uptake, VO_2 max) and muscular flexibility were evaluated using the Rockport fitness walking test [35] and the Bending test (executed from vertical and horizontal position) [36], respectively.

2.6. Statistical Analysis

An analysis of variance was performed to check any differences in baseline values (T0) among the 4 subgroups. Table 1 presented the mean values for the entire sample and for each group of exercise.

To evaluate the effects of the two forms of exercise programs, parameters at baseline and after three months of the exercise interventions were compared for each group through *t*-test for paired samples. Delta (Δ) changes (T1-T0) are presented as means and standard deviations (SDs).

Finally, to compare the NW and GYM exercise program effects, an analysis of variance of Δ changes (T1-T0) was performed. *p* values ≤ 0.05 were set as statistically significant. All the data have been digitally archived and the analyses were performed using SPSS® Software, version 22.0 (IBM Corp. Released 2013. IBM SPSS Statistics for Windows, Version 22.0. Armonk, NY: IBM Corp).

3. Results

One hundred and eight obese subjects were involved. All of them completed the entire exercise program and no side effects or injury were recorded. The rate of participation to the training sessions was 19.90 ± 4.28 out of 24 total sessions. The general percentage of adherence to both the exercise programs was 80.68 ± 14.47. Moreover, higher percentage of adherence to the GYM (OB-GYM = 87.22 ± 9.45; DM2-GYM = 87.30 ± 10.35) compared to the NW program (OB-NW = 71.86 ± 14.82; DM2-NW = 75.58 ± 17.90) was observed.

In all of the four groups, a statistically significant reduction in BW, BMI, fat mass index, muscular flexibility in vertical position (vertical bending) and VO_2 max were observed. For more information, please see: Figure 2a,b and Supplementary Material (attached file: "Table S1. Post-intervention assessments").

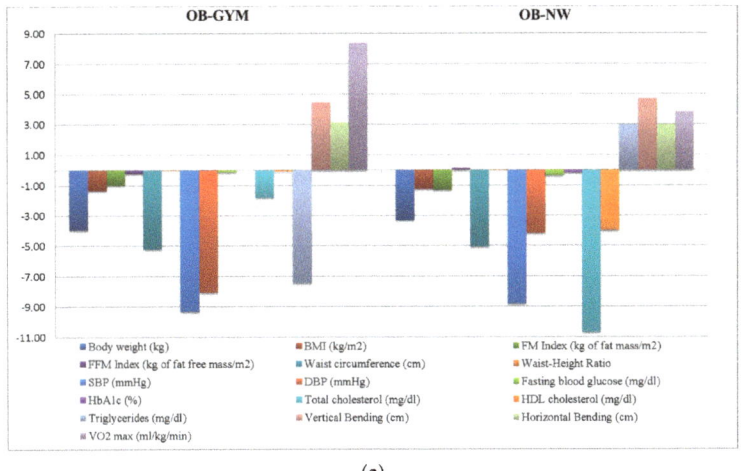

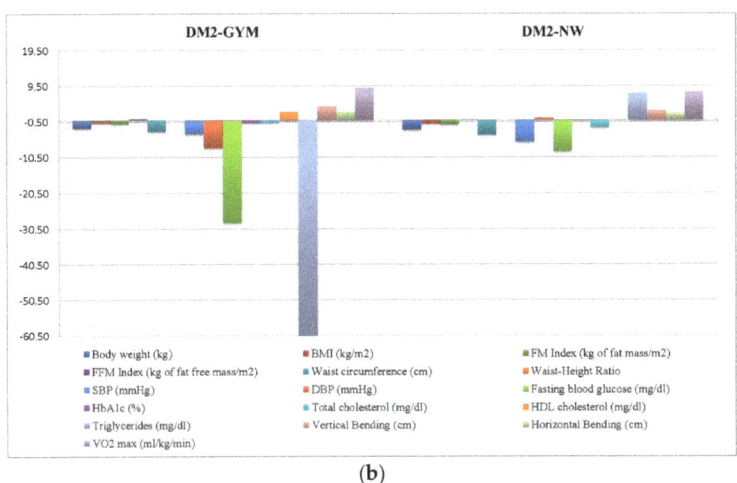

Figure 2. (**a**) Anthropometric profile, blood pressure levels, blood chemistry and fitness parameters in obese people. Results are presented as Δ (T1-T0) means. (**b**) Anthropometric profile, blood pressure levels, blood chemistry and fitness parameters in people with type 2 diabetes. Results are presented as Δ (T1-T0) means. Abbreviations: **OB-GYM**: individuals with obesity participating at gym-based exercise program; **OB-NW**: individuals with obesity participating at the Nordic walking exercise program; **DM2-GYM**: obese individuals with DM2 participating at the gym-based exercise program; **DM2-NW**: obese individuals with DM2 participating at the Nordic walking program.

In individuals with obesity only, significant improvements in BW, BMI, fat mass index, WC, WHR, vertical bending values, VO_2 max (all, $p < 0.01$) and systolic BP levels ($p = 0.01$) were found at the end of both exercise programs. Notably, only the OB-NW group showed significant improvements in HbA1c values ($p < 0.01$), total and HDL cholesterol levels ($p = 0.01$).

In obese individuals with DM2, significant improvements in BW, BMI, fat mass index, vertical bending results and VO_2 max levels were observed after both exercise programs. In addition, the DM2-GYM group showed significant improvements also in diastolic BP values ($p = 0.01$) and in the horizontal bending results ($p = 0.04$). In obese and diabetic individuals, the NW program allowed us to reach significant improvements also in WC and WHR ($p \leq 0.01$) measurements. In the

DM2-GYM group, we observed an important improvement in fasting blood glucose (−28.80 mg/dL) and triglycerides (−60.50 mg/dL). However, probably due to the small size of the sample, a significant statistic was not achieved. Overall, we found a significant relationship between proportional changes in plasma triglycerides and glucose metabolism after the program. In fact, proportional changes in plasma triglycerides explained 30% and 78% of the changes in plasma glucose and HbA1c, respectively. For more information please see Supplementary Materials (Table S2a and S2b).

4. Discussion

The aim of the study was to compare the cardiometabolic effects of two different supervised exercise programs (NW vs. GYM), following a multidisciplinary intervention performed at the C.U.R.I.A.Mo. center. Both exercise programs were developed in accordance with the ACSM guidelines for exercise testing and prescription in people with DM2 [28]. All participants completed the program and no side effects were recorded; this result suggested that, if the training program is developed following the guidelines, NW and GYM are two safe training modalities for obese patients with or without DM2 [37,38].

The promotion of general physical activity for health purposes, in the context of multidisciplinary lifestyle interventions, is essential to contrast sedentary lifestyle, which in turn contributes to an increase in the incidence of obesity and many other kinds of non-communicable chronic diseases [39]. Moreover, it was well-established that different forms of exercise-based interventions are strongly recommended in DM2 management [40]. In fact, the American Diabetes Association and the European Association for the Study of Diabetes stated that aerobic exercise, and the combination of aerobic exercise plus resistance training may be more effective than resistance training alone [41]. Structured and supervised exercise programs involving individuals with DM2 have been shown to be effective in antiatherogenic positive changes and in improving cardiometabolic parameters [5,42]. The C.U.R.I.A.Mo. multidisciplinary intervention already demonstrated encouraging results in obese subjects for some metabolic parameters [43], and in the glycemic control of those individuals with DM2 [44]. However, our findings reinforced the key role played by structured and supervised forms of exercise in DM2 management, underlining the therapeutic usefulness of non-conventional approaches, as is the case of NW training. Furthermore, our study compared two different forms of supervised exercise programs, providing an innovative message: in addition to the best-known conventional exercise-based therapies, special populations can choose among different types of validated approaches to exercise, according to their attitudes, motivations and interests.

As demonstrated by the findings of the UK Prospective Diabetes Study (UKPDS) [45], the positive changes in some cardiovascular risk factors and metabolic parameters resulted in a significant modification of the general cardiovascular risk score, crucial for increasing long-term cardiovascular protection. In obese and DM2 exercise groups, this study demonstrated the efficacy of both gym-based and NW exercise to improve BW, WC, BMI and fat mass index parameters. In this line, our findings show that in obese adults, a reduction in WHR measures was detected. Such element is closely connected with the decrease in general cardiovascular risk profile. Furthermore, the improvement in cardiorespiratory fitness (VO$_2$ max values) has been shown to be associated with a reduced total and cardiovascular mortality [46], both in the general and in the DM2 population [47]. Indeed, some of the previous studies [48,49] reported that increases of approximately 3.5 mL/min/kg in VO$_2$ max values are associated with a reduction in all-cause mortality superior to 10%. In our study, increments of VO$_2$ max have shown to reach values superior to these data [48,49] (GYM groups: 8.38 and 9.06; NW groups: 3.83 and 7.9), supporting the strong need to comprise the therapeutic exercise within the multidisciplinary care of populations with metabolic diseases.

Although many studies showed that the exercise performed in a natural environment determines greater adherence [50–53], our findings registered an opposite result. According to other authors [54–56], it is possible that individuals, who participated at the NW program, being mainly women, meet multiple barriers to assure a continuative exercise participation, such as lack of time (e.g., due to household tasks) and feelings of guilt. Despite the lower adherence (−14.4%), the NW program determined the same positive responses to GYM in individuals with DM2. Furthermore, in the obese individuals NW determined a greater reduction in metabolic values. This could indicate that NW has a greater cardiometabolic efficacy than the GYM program, likely due to the continuous active use of muscles of trunk, upper and lower limbs.

In their study [57,58], Balducci et al. reported that there is not yet conclusive evidence that positive changes in physical activity levels can be sustained over the long term, however, our study highlighted that supervised exercise programs can support patients' adherence to exercise-based treatment, recording a general activities participation of 80.7%. According to Italian [25] and ACSM/ADA [26] guidelines, our results support the recommendation for qualified exercise-trainer supervision (graduate sports science specialists), both to minimize risk of injuries and overall to achieve tailored health aims that are capable of effectively counteracting such kinds of non-communicable diseases from spreading worldwide. Other authors have shown that unsupervised NW trainings seem to not fulfill enough increase in exercise intensity in order to achieve those health advantages specific to individuals with DM2 [59]. From this point of view, for those subjects belonging to special populations who choose to carry out unconventional therapeutic exercise-based activities such as NW, aquatic exercise and other fitness workouts, it is imperative to follow the main guidelines on exercise prescription and be supported by the guidance of exercise science specialists for the entire duration of tailored exercise programs [60,61].

5. Conclusions

Our findings show that a supervised NW program is as effective as a conventional GYM program in improving BW control, body composition, muscular flexibility and VO_2 max levels in obese adults with and without DM2; notwithstanding, we recorded a significantly lower adherence to NW than GYM programs. Furthermore, NW is an easy-to-learn activity performable in different environments, rarely associated with physical injuries, more adaptable than GYM with regard to lack of time, low fitness level, and shortage of money, requiring only specific poles. This allows us to state the major efficacy of NW over GYM program, in improving cardiometabolic parameters of both obese people with and without DM2. However, the lack of a normal-weight control group did not permit a deepened knowledge of the effects of NW and GYM programs on cardiometabolic parameters in obese subjects with and without DM2. Ultimately, our study emphasizes the awareness that in addition to the best-known conventional exercise-based therapies, populations with metabolic diseases can opt also to do other forms of validated exercises according to their attitudes, motivations and interests.

Supplementary Materials: The following are available online at http://www.mdpi.com/2411-5142/5/3/62/s1, Table S1: Post-intervention assessments; Table S2a and S2b: Descriptive statistics and Delta changes of plasma triglycerides and glucose metabolism correlations.

Author Contributions: Conceptualization, R.P., C.A. and L.C.; methodology, R.P., C.A. and C.F.; validation, R.P., C.A. and C.F.; formal analysis, C.A., R.P. and A.D.B.; investigation, C.A. and R.P.; resources C.F.; data curation, C.A., R.P. and A.D.B.; writing—original draft preparation, R.P., C.A., A.D.B., V.B., S.G., M.B. and L.C.; writing—review and editing, R.P., C.A., C.F., A.D.B., V.B., S.G., M.B. and L.C.; supervision, C.F. R.P., M.B., and L.C.; project administration, C.F. and R.P.; funding acquisition, C.F. All authors have read and agreed to the published version of the manuscript.

Funding: This research received no external funding.

Acknowledgments: The Centro Universitario Ricerca Interdipartimentale Attività Motoria project is supported by a grant from the Department of Health of the Umbria Region (Italy).

Conflicts of Interest: The authors declare no conflict of interest. The funders had no role in the design of the study; in the collection, analyses, or interpretation of data; in the writing of the manuscript, or in the decision to publish the results.

References

1. Stamatakis, E.; Gale, J.; Bauman, A.; Ekelund, U.; Hamer, M.; Ding, D. Sitting Time, Physical Activity, and Risk of Mortality in Adults. *J. Am. Coll. Cardiol.* **2019**, *73*, 2062–2072. [CrossRef] [PubMed]
2. International Diabetes Federation. IDF Diabetes Atlas 2019. Available online: https://www.diabetesatlas.org/upload/resources/2019/IDF_Atlas_9th_Edition_2019.pdf (accessed on 1 March 2019).
3. De Feo, P.; Di Loreto, C.; Ranchelli, A.; Fatone, C.; Gambelunghe, G.; Lucidi, P.; Santeusanio, F. Exercise and diabetes. *Acta Biomed.* **2006**, *77*, 14–17. [PubMed]
4. Horton, E.S. Role and management of exercise in diabetes mellitus. *Diabetes Care* **1988**, *11*, 201–211. [CrossRef] [PubMed]
5. Umpierre, D.; Ribeiro, P.A.; Kramer, C.K.; Leitao, C.B.; Zucatti, A.T.; Azevedo, M.J.; Gross, J.L.; Ribeiro, J.P.; Schaan, B.D. Physical activity advice only or structured exercise training and association with HbA1c levels in type 2 diabetes: A systematic review and meta-analysis. *JAMA* **2011**, *305*, 1790–1799. [CrossRef] [PubMed]
6. Marini, E.; Mariani, P.G.; Ministrini, S.; Pippi, R.; Aiello, C.; Reginato, E.; Siepi, D.; Innocente, S.; Lombardini, R.; Paltriccia, R.; et al. Combined aerobic and resistance training improves microcirculation in metabolic syndrome. *J. Sports Med. Phys. Fit.* **2019**, *59*, 1571–1576. [CrossRef]
7. Fatone, C.; Guescini, M.; Balducci, S.; Battistoni, S.; Settequattrini, A.; Pippi, R.; Stocchi, L.; Mantuano, M.; Stocchi, V.; De Feo, P. Two weekly sessions of combined aerobic and resistance exercise are sufficient to provide beneficial effects in subjects with Type 2 diabetes mellitus and metabolic syndrome. *J. Endocrinol. Investig.* **2010**, *33*, 489–495. [CrossRef]
8. Boule, N.G.; Kenny, G.P.; Haddad, E.; Wells, G.A.; Sigal, R.J. Meta-analysis of the effect of structured exercise training on cardiorespiratory fitness in Type 2 diabetes mellitus. *Diabetologia* **2003**, *46*, 1071–1081.
9. Yaribeygi, H.; Butler, A.E.; Sahebkar, A. Aerobic exercise can modulate the underlying mechanisms involved in the development of diabetic complications. *J. Cell. Physiol.* **2019**, *234*, 12508–12515. [CrossRef]
10. Rachel, S.; Denise, S. The benefits of regular walking for health, well-being and the environment. *C3 Collab. Health.* September 2012. Available online: https://www.c3health.org/wp-content/uploads/2017/07/C3-report-on-walking-v-1-20120911.pdf (accessed on 1 May 2019).
11. Katsanos, C.S. Prescribing aerobic exercise for the regulation of postprandial lipid metabolism: Current research and recommendations. *Sports Med.* **2006**, *36*, 547–560. [CrossRef]
12. Slentz, C.A.; Aiken, L.B.; Houmard, J.A.; Bales, C.W.; Johnson, J.L.; Tanner, C.J.; Duscha, B.D.; Kraus, W.E. Inactivity, exercise, and visceral fat. STRRIDE: A randomized, controlled study of exercise intensity and amount. *J. Appl. Physiol.* **2005**, *99*, 1613–1618. [CrossRef]
13. De Feo, P. Is high-intensity exercise better than moderate-intensity exercise for weight loss? *Nutr. Metab. Cardiovasc. Dis.* **2013**, *23*, 1037–1042. [CrossRef] [PubMed]
14. Schiffer, T.; Knicker, A.; Hoffman, U.; Harwig, B.; Hollmann, W.; Strüder, H.K. Physiological responses to nordic walking, walking and jogging. *Eur. J. Appl. Physiol.* **2006**, *98*, 56–61. [CrossRef] [PubMed]
15. Hansen, E.A.; Smith, G. Energy expenditure and comfort during Nordic walking with different pole lengths. *J. Strength Cond. Res.* **2009**, *23*, 1187–1194. [CrossRef]
16. Cugusi, L.; Manca, A.; Dragone, D.; Deriu, F.; Solla, P.; Secci, C.; Monticone, M.; Mercuro, G. Nordic Walking for the Management of People With Parkinson Disease: A Systematic Review. *PM R* **2017**, *9*, 1157–1166. [CrossRef]
17. Bullo, V.; Gobbo, S.; Vendramin, B.; Duregon, F.; Cugusi, L.; Di Blasio, A.; Bocalini, D.S.; Zaccaria, M.; Bergamin, M.; Ermolao, A. Nordic Walking Can Be Incorporated in the Exercise Prescription to Increase Aerobic Capacity, Strength, and Quality of Life for Elderly: A Systematic Review and Meta-Analysis. *Rejuvenation Res.* **2018**, *21*, 141–161. [CrossRef] [PubMed]
18. Cugusi, L.; Manca, A.; Yeo, T.J.; Bassareo, P.P.; Mercuro, G.; Kaski, J.C. Nordic walking for individuals with cardiovascular disease: A systematic review and meta-analysis of randomized controlled trials. *Eur. J. Prev. Cardiol.* **2017**, *24*, 1938–1955. [CrossRef] [PubMed]
19. Gobbo, S.; Bullo, V.; Roma, E.; Duregon, F.; Bocalini, D.S.; Rica, R.L.; Di Blasio, A.; Cugusi, L.; Vendramin, B.; Bergamo, M.; et al. Nordic Walking Promoted Weight Loss in Overweight and Obese People: A Systematic Review for Future Exercise Prescription. *J. Funct. Morphol. Kinesiol.* **2019**, *4*, 36. [CrossRef]
20. Vilchez Barrera, M.; Calvo-Arencibia, A. Scientific evidence of nordic walking in Physiotherapy: Bibliographic review. *Fisioterapia* **2016**, *38*, 251–264.

21. Sentinelli, F.; La Cava, V.; Serpe, R.O.B.E.R.T.O.; Boi, A.; Incani, M.I.C.H.E.L.A.; Manconi, E.T.T.O.R.E.; Solinas, A.L.D.O.; Cossu, E.; Lenzi, A.; Baroni, M.G. Positive effects of Nordic Walking on anthropometric and metabolic variables in women with type 2 diabetes mellitus. *Sci. Sports* **2015**, *30*, 25–32. [CrossRef]
22. Fritz, T.; Caidahl, K.; Krook, A.; Lundström, P.; Mashili, F.; Osler, M.; Szekeres, F.L.; Östenson, C.G.; Wändell, P.; Zierath, J.R. Effects of Nordic walking on cardiovascular risk factors in overweight individuals with type 2 diabetes, impaired or normal glucose tolerance. *Diabetes Metab. Res. Rev.* **2013**, *29*, 25–32. [CrossRef]
23. Gram, B.; Christensen, R.; Christiansen, C.; Gram, J. Effects of nordic walking and exercise in type 2 diabetes mellitus: A randomized controlled trial. *Clin. J. Sport. Med.* **2010**, *20*, 355–361. [PubMed]
24. De Feo, P.; Fatone, C.; Burani, P.; Piana, N.; Pazzagli, C.; Battistini, D.; Capezzali, D.; Pippi, R.; Chipi, B.; Mazzeschi, C. An innovative model for changing the lifestyles of persons with obesity and/or Type 2 diabetes mellitus. *J. Endocrinol. Investig.* **2011**, *34*, e349–e354. [PubMed]
25. (AMD) A.M.D.; S.I.d.D. (SID). *Standard Italiani Per La Cura Del Diabete Mellito 2018*; Available online: http://www.siditalia.it/pdf/Standard%20di%20Cura%20AMD%20-%20SID%202018_protetto2.pdf (accessed on 1 February 2019).
26. Colberg, S.R.; Sigal, R.J.; Fernhall, B.; Regensteiner, J.G.; Blissmer, B.J.; Rubin, R.R.; Chasan-Taber, L.; Albright, A.L.; Braun, B. Exercise and type 2 diabetes: The American College of Sports Medicine and the American Diabetes Association: Joint position statement. *Diabetes Care* **2010**, *33*, e147–e167. [CrossRef] [PubMed]
27. Balducci, S.; Zanuso, S.; Massarini, M.; Corigliano, G.; Nicolucci, A.; Missori, S.; Cavallo, S.; Cardelli, P.; Alessi, E.; Pugliese, G.; et al. The Italian Diabetes and Exercise Study (IDES): Design and methods for a prospective Italian multicentre trial of intensive lifestyle intervention in people with type 2 diabetes and the metabolic syndrome. *Nutr. Metab. Cardiovasc. Dis.* **2008**, *18*, 585–595. [CrossRef]
28. American College of Sports, Medicine; Riebe, D.; Ehrman, J.K.; Liguori, G.; Magal, M. *ACSM's Guidelines for Exercise Testing and Prescription*; Wolters Kluwer: Philadelphia, PA, USA, 2018.
29. Karvonen, J.; Vuorimaa, T. Heart rate and exercise intensity during sports activities. Practical application. *Sports Med.* **1988**, *5*, 303–311. [CrossRef]
30. Brzycki, M. Strength Testing—Predicting a One-Rep Max from Reps-to-Fatigue. *J. Phys. Edication Recreat. Danc.* **1993**, *64*, 88–90. [CrossRef]
31. Habicht, J.P. Standardization of quantitative epidemiological methods in the field. *Bol. Oficina Sani. Panam.* **1974**, *76*, 375–384.
32. VanItallie, T.B.; Yang, M.U.; Heymsfield, S.B.; Funk, R.C.; Boileau, R.A. Height-normalized indices of the body's fat-free mass and fat mass: Potentially useful indicators of nutritional status. *Am. J. Clin. Nutr.* **1990**, *52*, 953–959. [CrossRef]
33. Ashwell, M.; Gunn, P.; Gibson, S. Waist-to-height ratio is a better screening tool than waist circumference and BMI for adult cardiometabolic risk factors: Systematic review and meta-analysis. *Obes. Rev.* **2012**, *13*, 275–286. [CrossRef]
34. Linares, C.L.; Ciangura, C.; Bouillot, J.L.; Coupaye, M.; Declèves, X.; Poitou, C.; Basdevant, A.; Oppert, J.M. Validity of leg-to-leg bioelectrical impedance analysis to estimate body fat in obesity. *Obes. Surg.* **2011**, *21*, 917–923. [CrossRef]
35. Weiglein, L.; Herrick, J.; Kirk, S.; Kirk, E.P. The 1-mile walk test is a valid predictor of VO_{2max} and is a reliable alternative fitness test to the 1.5-mile run in US Air Force males. *Mil. Med.* **2011**, *176*, 669–673. [CrossRef] [PubMed]
36. Mayorga-Vega, D.; Merino-Marban, R.; Viciana, J. Criterion-Related Validity of Sit-and-Reach Tests for Estimating Hamstring and Lumbar Extensibility: A Meta-Analysis. *J. Sports. Sci. Med.* **2014**, *13*, 1–14. [PubMed]
37. Kucio, C.; Narloch, D.; Kucio, E.; Kurek, J. The application of Nordic walking in the treatment hypertension and obesity. *Fam. Med. Prim. Care Rev.* **2017**, *19*, 144–148. [CrossRef]
38. Venojarvi, M.; Wasenius, N.; Manderoos, S.; Heinonen, O.J.; Hernelahti, M.; Lindholm, H.; Surakka, J.; Lindström, J.; Aunola, S.; Atalay, M.; et al. Nordic walking decreased circulating chemerin and leptin concentrations in middle-aged men with impaired glucose regulation. *Ann. Med.* **2013**, *45*, 162–170. [CrossRef]

39. Jain, R.; Olejas, S.; Feh, A.R.; Edwards, A.; Abigo, I.; Zietek, W.; Khan, Z.; Ragoonanan, S.; Benoy, N.; Bramble, D. Review the evidence for lifestyle management in the prevention of type 2 diabetes and compare them to pharmacological interventions. *EC Diabetes Metab. Res.* **2020**, *4*, 161–166. [CrossRef]
40. Ried-Larsen, M.; MacDonald, C.S.; Johansen, M.Y.; Hansen, K.B.; Christensen, R.; Almdal, T.P.; Pedersen, B.K.; Karstoft, K. Why prescribe exercise as therapy in type 2 diabetes? We have a pill for that! *Diabetes Metab. Res. Rev.* **2018**, *34*, e2999. [CrossRef]
41. Davies, M.J.; D'Alessio, D.A.; Fradkin, J.; Kernan, W.N.; Mathieu, C.; Mingrone, G.; Rossing, P.; Tsapas, A.; Wexler, D.J.; Buse, J.B. Management of Hyperglycemia in Type 2 Diabetes, 2018. A Consensus Report by the American Diabetes Association (ADA) and the European Association for the Study of Diabetes (EASD). *Diabetes Care* **2018**, *41*, 2669–2701. [CrossRef]
42. Johansen, M.Y.; MacDonald, C.S.; Hansen, K.B.; Karstoft, K.; Christensen, R.; Pedersen, M.; Hansen, L.S.; Zacho, M.; Wedell-Neergaard, A.S.; Nielsen, S.T.; et al. Effect of an Intensive Lifestyle Intervention on Glycemic Control in Patients With Type 2 Diabetes: A Randomized Clinical Trial. *JAMA* **2017**, *318*, 637–646. [CrossRef]
43. Russo, A.; Pirisinu, I.; Vacca, C.; Reginato, E.; Tomaro, E.S.; Pippi, R.; Aiello, C.; Talesa, V.N.; De Feo, P.; Romani, R. An intensive lifestyle intervention reduces circulating oxidised low-density lipoprotein and increases human paraoxonase activity in obese subjects. *Obes. Res. Clin. Pract.* **2018**, *12*, 108–114. [CrossRef]
44. Tomaro, E.S.; Pippi, R.; Reginato, E.; Aiello, C.; Buratta, L.; Mazzeschi, C.; Perrone, C.; Ranucci, C.; Tirimagni, A.; Russo, A.; et al. Intensive lifestyle intervention is particularly advantageous in poorly controlled type 2 diabetes. *Nutr. Metab. Cardiovasc. Dis.* **2017**, *27*, 688–694. [CrossRef]
45. Holman, R.R.; Paul, S.K.; Bethel, M.A.; Matthews, D.R.; Neil, H.A.W. 10-year follow-up of intensive glucose control in type 2 diabetes. *N. Engl. J. Med.* **2008**, *359*, 1577–1589. [CrossRef] [PubMed]
46. Blair, S.N.; Kampert, J.B.; Kohl, H.W.; Barlow, C.E.; Macera, C.A.; Paffenbarger, R.S.; Gibbons, L.W. Influences of cardiorespiratory fitness and other precursors on cardiovascular disease and all-cause mortality in men and women. *JAMA* **1996**, *276*, 205–210. [CrossRef] [PubMed]
47. Church, T.S.; Cheng, Y.J.; Earnest, C.P.; Barlow, C.E.; Gibbons, L.W.; Priest, E.L.; Blair, S.N. Exercise capacity and body composition as predictors of mortality among men with diabetes. *Diabetes Care* **2004**, *27*, 83–88. [CrossRef] [PubMed]
48. Kokkinos, P.; Myers, J.; Nylen, E.; Panagiotakos, D.B.; Manolis, A.; Pittaras, A.; Blackman, M.R.; Jacob-Issac, R.; Faselis, C.; Abella, J.; et al. Exercise capacity and all-cause mortality in African American and Caucasian men with type 2 diabetes. *Diabetes Care* **2009**, *32*, 623–628. [CrossRef]
49. Ross, R.; Blair, S.N.; Arena, R.; Church, T.S.; Després, J.P.; Franklin, B.A.; Haskell, W.L.; Kaminsky, L.A.; Levine, B.D.; Lavie, C.J.; et al. Importance of Assessing Cardiorespiratory Fitness in Clinical Practice: A Case for Fitness as a Clinical Vital Sign: A Scientific Statement From the American Heart Association. *Circulation* **2016**, *134*, e653–e699. [CrossRef]
50. Lahart, I.; Darcy, P.; Gidlow, C.; Calogiuri, G. The Effects of Green Exercise on Physical and Mental Wellbeing: A Systematic Review. *Int. J. Environ. Res. Public Health* **2019**, *16*, 1352. [CrossRef]
51. McArthur, D.; Dumas, A.; Woodend, K.; Beach, S.; Stacey, D. Factors influencing adherence to regular exercise in middle-aged women: A qualitative study to inform clinical practice. *BMC Womens Health* **2014**, *14*, 49. [CrossRef]
52. Gladwell, V.F.; Brown, D.K.; Wood, C.; Sandercock, G.R.; Barton, J.L. The great outdoors: How a green exercise environment can benefit all. *Extrem. Physiol. Med.* **2013**, *2*, 3. [CrossRef]
53. Fluery-Bahi, G.; Pol, E.; Navarro, O. International Handbooks of Quality-of-life. In *Handbook of Environmental Psychology and Quality of Life Research*, 1st ed.; Springer International Publishing: Cham, Switzerland, 2017; Volume XIII, p. 574.
54. Hoare, E.; Stavreski, B.; Jennings, G.L.; Kingwell, B.A. Exploring Motivation and Barriers to Physical Activity among Active and Inactive Australian Adults. *Sports* **2017**, *5*, 47. [CrossRef]
55. Moreno, J.; Johnson, C. Barriers to physical activity in women. *Am. J. Lifestyle Med.* **2014**, *8*, 164–166. [CrossRef]
56. Eyler, A.E.; Wilcox, S.; Matson-Koffman, D.; Evenson, K.R.; Sanderson, B.; Thompson, J.; Wilbur, J.; Rohm-Young, D. Correlates of physical activity among women from diverse racial/ethnic groups. *J. Womens Health Gend. Based Med.* **2002**, *11*, 239–253. [CrossRef] [PubMed]

57. Balducci, S.; D'Errico, V.; Haxhi, J.; Sacchetti, M.; Orlando, G.; Cardelli, P.; Vitale, M.; Bollanti, L.; Conti, F.; Zanuso, S.; et al. Effect of a Behavioral Intervention Strategy on Sustained Change in Physical Activity and Sedentary Behavior in Patients With Type 2 Diabetes: The IDES_2 Randomized Clinical Trial. *JAMA* **2019**, *321*, 880–890. [CrossRef] [PubMed]
58. Balducci, S.; Zanuso, S.; Nicolucci, A.; De Feo, P.; Cavallo, S.; Cardelli, P.; Fallucca, S.; Alessi, E.; Fallucca, F.; Pugliese, G. Effect of an intensive exercise intervention strategy on modifiable cardiovascular risk factors in subjects with type 2 diabetes mellitus: A randomized controlled trial: The Italian Diabetes and Exercise Study (IDES). *Arch. Intern. Med.* **2010**, *170*, 1794–1803. [CrossRef] [PubMed]
59. Fritz, T.; Caidahl, K.; Osler, M.; Östenson, C.G.; Zierath, J.R.; Wändell, P. Effects of Nordic walking on health-related quality of life in overweight individuals with type 2 diabetes mellitus, impaired or normal glucose tolerance. *Diabet. Med.* **2011**, *28*, 1362–1372. [CrossRef]
60. Cugusi, L.; Manca, A.; Bassareo, P.P.; Crisafulli, A.; Deriu, F.; Mercuro, G. Supervised aquatic-based exercise for men with coronary artery disease: A meta-analysis of randomised controlled trials. *Eur. J. Prev. Cardiol.* **2019**, 1–6. [CrossRef] [PubMed]
61. Cugusi, L.; Cadeddu, C.; Nocco, S.; Orrù, F.; Bandino, S.; Deidda, M.; Caria, A.; Bassareo, P.P.; Piras, A.; Cabras, S.; et al. Effects of an aquatic-based exercise program to improve cardiometabolic profile, quality of life, and physical activity levels in men with type 2 diabetes mellitus. *PM R* **2015**, *7*, 141–148. [CrossRef]

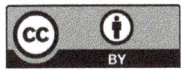

© 2020 by the authors. Licensee MDPI, Basel, Switzerland. This article is an open access article distributed under the terms and conditions of the Creative Commons Attribution (CC BY) license (http://creativecommons.org/licenses/by/4.0/).

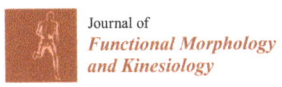

Journal of
Functional Morphology and Kinesiology

Article

Effects of Different Resistance Training Frequencies on Body Composition, Cardiometabolic Risk Factors, and Handgrip Strength in Overweight and Obese Women: A Randomized Controlled Trial

Francesco Campa [1], Pasqualino Maietta Latessa [2], Gianpiero Greco [3], Mario Mauro [3,*], Paolo Mazzuca [4], Federico Spiga [1] and Stefania Toselli [1]

[1] Department of Biomedical and Neuromotor Sciences, University of Bologna, 40126 Bologna, Italy; francesco.campa3@unibo.it (F.C.); Federico2907@gmail.com (F.S.); stefania.toselli@unibo.it (S.T.)
[2] Department for Life Quality Studies, University of Bologna, 47921 Rimini, Italy; pasqualino.maietta@unibo.it
[3] Department of Basic Medical Sciences, Neuroscience and Sense Organs, University of Study of Bari, 70121 Bari, Italy; gianpierogreco.phd@yahoo.com
[4] Unit of Internal Medicine, Diabetes and Metabolic Disease Center, Romagna Health District, 47921 Rimini, Italy; Paolo.mazzuca4@unibo.it
* Correspondence: mario.mauro.194@gmail.com; Tel.: +39-3388259249

Received: 26 May 2020; Accepted: 15 July 2020; Published: 17 July 2020

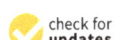

Abstract: Background: Resistance training improves health in obese and overweight people. However, it is not clear what is the optimal weekly resistance training frequency and the most efficacious training protocol on body composition, cardiometabolic risk factors, and handgrip strength (HS). The aim of this study was to determine the effects of a supervised structured 24 week resistance training program on obese and overweight women. Methods: Forty-five women (BMI 37.1 ± 6.3 kg/m^2; age 56.5 ± 0.7 years) were randomly assigned to one of two groups: A group with a high weekly training frequency of three times a week (HIGH) and a group that performed it only once a week (LOW). Cardiometabolic risk factors, anthropometric and HS measures were taken before and after the intervention period. Results: A significant ($p < 0.05$) group by time interaction was observed for body weight, body mass index, waist circumference, fat mass, plasma glucose, plasma insulin, homeostatic model assessment, and for dominant and absolute HS. Additionally, only the HIGH group saw increased HS and decreased total cholesterol and LDL-cholesterol after the intervention period ($p < 0.05$). The observed increase in HS was associated with an improved insulin resistance sensitivity (absolute handgrip strength: $r = -0.40$, $p = 0.007$; relative handgrip strength: $r = -0.47$, $p = 0.001$) after training, which constitutes an essential element for cardiovascular health. Conclusions: The results suggest that high weekly frequency training give greater benefits for weight loss and cardiometabolic risk factors improvement than a training program with a training session of once a week. Furthermore, the improvement of HS can be achieved with a high weekly frequency training.

Keywords: body weight; obesity; physical activity

1. Introduction

Overweight and obesity are major risk factors for a number of chronic diseases, including cardiovascular diseases such as heart disease and stroke, which are the leading causes of death worldwide [1]. According to the 1998 overweight and obesity clinical guidelines, overweight is defined as a BMI ranging from 25 to 29.9 kg/m^2 and obesity as a BMI ≥ 30 kg/m^2 [2]. From 1999–2000 to 2017–2018, the age-adjusted prevalence of obesity increased from 30.5% to 42.4%, and the prevalence of severe obesity increased from 4.7% to 9.2% in the USA [3]. In addition, the overall prevalence of obesity was similar among men and women, but the prevalence of severe obesity was higher among women and adults aged 40–59 [3]. In 2017, 52% of adults worldwide and 65% of adults in the UK were classified as overweight or obese [4]. Moreover, in most of Northern European and Southern European countries, the rate of obesity has doubled in the last 30 years [5,6].

Obesity is correlated with morphological changes resulting from an increased deposition of lipid within muscle fibers, which decreases muscle quality and contributes to frailty by reducing muscle strength and increasing disability [7]. The high percentage of overweight/obese people with the poor metabolic control of diabetes has become an important public health problem in recent years [8–10]. Although bariatric surgery is the most effective treatment to reduce and maintain weight loss [11,12], another effective strategy is represented by a lifestyle modification that includes a prescription for increased physical activity [13,14].

A weight change of 3% to 5% may lead to clinically meaningful health benefits and losing 5% to 10% of weight can decrease the cardiovascular risk factor, morbidity, and mortality [15,16]. Resistance training is a physical activity which promotes improvements in body composition and most cardiometabolic risk factors [17,18]. It can reduce blood pressure, total cholesterol and plasma triglycerides, inducing beneficial effects on circulating inflammatory markers and reducing insulin resistance sensitivity [19–21]. In addition, enhancements in body composition are associated to a better quality of life [22]. Resistance exercise is also effective to increase muscular strength [23,24], especially that of handgrip [25,26].

Recent studies, which have offered resistance training as a physical activity for obese and overweight people, have used training protocols with a frequency of two or three times a week [27,28]. Studies on training frequency in older adults have shown different results, with some reporting no differences between lower and higher frequencies on muscle mass [29,30], while others have reported that muscle strength and functional performance are favored with higher frequencies [31,32]. However, to our knowledge, no study compared the effects of different resistance training frequencies on the most informative parameters of the health status in obese and overweight people.

Therefore, the aim of this study was to compare the effects of a resistance training program of one or three times a week on body composition, cardiometabolic risk factors, and handgrip strength in overweight and obese women. We hypothesized that a higher training frequency could have a better impact on the examined parameters, especially on handgrip strength development.

2. Materials and Methods

2.1. Participants

To identify the sample size for the study, we assessed an a "priori: computer required sample size-given α, power and Effect Size" by G*Power (3.1.9.2, Üversität Kiel, Germany). A repeated measures ANOVA was selected as the F test of all the test family, inputing the following parameters: α = 0.05; (1−β) = 0.8; Effect Size f = 0.5. The outcomes parameters thus calculated detected a sample size of 19 participants for each group, totalling 38 participants. To meet this, we estimated a follow-up loss rate of about 10 people and selected 50 subjects who were women aged 56.5 ± 8.7 years and with a BMI 37.1 ± 6.3 kg/m^2. They were chosen from the Lifestyle program of the "Infermi" Endocrinology Department (Rimini) and voluntarily participated in our study. To comply with our treatment inclusion criteria, the participants could not have a body mass index ≤ 25 kg/m^2. To prevent the affected outcomes they were not to smoke, were not to take medications and they did not have any major disease (cardiovascular disease, etc.). In addition, they had not participated in a physical exercise program over the last six months before the study. Menopausal status and menstrual cycle info were collected during two interviews before the tests, as previously stated by our group [33].

A randomized controlled trial was conducted for up to 28 weeks, of which 4 (first, second, second to last and last) were employed for assessment and measurements and 24 weeks were used for the exercise treatment. The participants were randomly allocated to each group following the study purpose: An experimental group who performed the exercise program with a weekly frequency of three times per week (HIGH) and a control group who performed the exercise program just once per week (LOW). The participants were recommended did not eat for at least two hours before the exercise program. The random allocation (random.org) was carried out by a blinded researcher. Different places were selected for measurements, which were assessed in the hospital department, and exercise which was performed in a contracted sports center. Our study followed the CONSORT statement recommendations for reporting randomized trials [32]. All participants provided their written, informed consent to participate after all procedures were explained. The study was approved by the Bioethics Committee of the University of Bologna and was conducted in accordance with the guidelines of the Declaration of Helsinki; project identification code was NCT03410329 (25 January 2018).

2.2. Exercise Program

The 24 week resistance training program was performed under the supervision of an exercise physiologist. During first two weeks, he exhibited how to execute each exercise correctly and theh participants had to familiarize with it. After this learning period, the exercise physiologist tested each participant workload at 10 repetitions for every exercise programmed. The resistance training program was about 65 min for both the exercise and the control group and for all of the experiment period. Exercise selection and sequence never changed over time and between groups. Workouts included an initial 10 min warm-up at low intensity (30–50% HRmax), performed using a treadmill, stepper, elliptical, or cycle ergometer, as preferred by the subjects. The central part of the program had a duration of 45 min and included seven exercises on isotonic machines with the specific sequence: leg extension and leg press for leg muscles, lat machine and low row for back muscles, pectoral machine and chest press for chest muscles and shoulder press for shoulder muscles. Following Ehrman and colleagues' recommendations for obese people [34], every exercise provided four sets of 8–12 repetitions in a range of 60–80% one repetition maximum (1-RM); each set was performed in about 30 s with 1 min of rest between series and 2 min of rest among exercises. Whenever the participants reached less than 8 repetitions, a decreased weight of 5% was advised to perform after a short rest; similarly, whether the participants reached more than 12 repetitions, an increased weight of 5% was required to perform after a short rest. In addition, to meet the basic principles of resistance training progression [35] every 2 weeks the exercise physiologist increased the intensity by 5% on a muscular group exercise (leg, back, chest or shoulder) and tested it on the participants: if they were able to perform it, the new workload was set, whereas if they were not able to perform it, the workload did not change. Finally, the participants performed 10 min of cool down on a treadmill at the same intensity of the initial warm-up. The HIGH group performed the training program on Monday, Wednesday and Friday evening (6 p.m.) with 48 h of rest between sessions; the LOW group performed the training program on Thursday evening.

2.3. Anthropometry

All the measurements were carried out by a physician specifically trained in physical anthropometry and blinded to group assignment. To calculate the BMI (kg/m^2) of each participant, we needed to evaluate the anthropometric features of height and weight. These were measured according to standard methods [36], using a stadiometer which recorded the height at an accuracy of 0.1 cm and a high-precision mechanical scale (Seca, Basel, Switzerland) for recording weight at an accuracy of 0.1 kg. Moreover, each participant's waist circumference (WC) was recorded. It was taken at the narrowest part of the torso [36]. Skinfold thicknesses at four sites (biceps, triceps, subscapular and suprailiac) were measured to the nearest 0.1 mm with a Lange skinfold caliper (Beta technology Inc., Cambridge, MD, USA). For each anthropometrical point considered, three non-consecutive measurements were performed in order to extract the average. The technical error of measurement scores (TEM) was required to be within 5% agreement for skinfolds and within 1% for WC. Skinfold values were used in anthropometric regression equations to predict fat mass [37,38].

2.4. Cardiometabolic Risk Factors

Routine laboratory testing was carried out in all cases at entry; plasma glucose, total cholesterol (TC), high-density lipoprotein (HDL) cholesterol, and triglycerides (TG) were measured with routine assays using internal and external quality controls. Low-density lipoprotein (LDL) cholesterol was calculated using the Friedewald formula [39]. The homeostasis model assessment ($HOMA_{IR}$), insulin resistance index, was calculated as the fasting plasma insulin concentration (mU/l) × fasting plasma glucose concentration (mmol/l)/22.5. Glycated hemoglobin (HbA1c) was measured by exchange high-performance liquid chromatograph using standardized laboratory procedures. Blood pressure was taken by an automatic monitor (Omron1 Model HEM-7011, Omron Healthcare, Inc., Bannockburn, IL, USA) three times successively with at least a one-minute interval between each reading. The average of the three blood pressure measurements was used for analysis.

2.5. Handgrip Strength

A mechanical dynamometer (Takei K.K. 5001, Takei Scientific Instruments, Ltd., Niigata City, Japan) was used to evaluate the left and right handgrip strengths at an accuracy of 0.5 kg to carry out the dominant (DHS) and absolute handgrip strength (AHS). Each participant was evaluated by keeping the dynamometer at a 90-degree flexion of their elbow, in a sitting position for a maximum of three attempts for each hand. The AHS was calculated as the sum of the right and left hand outcomes. Finally, the relative handgrip strength (RHS) was calculated following Choquette and colleagues [40], as the relationship between handgrip strength (HS) and BMI.

2.6. Statistical Analyses

Normality was checked with the Shapiro–Wilk test. The two-way ANOVA for between- and within-group comparisons was assessed to accept the main hypothesis. Bonferroni's post hoc test was employed to detect specific differences in the variables where the F-ratio was significant. A two-way repeated measures ANCOVA was assessed for comparisons with the covariates as age, weight loss, and menopausal status. Effect size (*ES*) was calculated as the difference between the post-training mean and the pre-training mean related to the pooled standard deviation [8]. The *ES* was classified as follows: it was considered as small when its value was 0.20–0.49, moderate when it was 0.50–0.79, and large when it was ≥0.80. To compare the changes in weight status categories after the intervention period, the McNemar test for paired proportions was used. Bivariate and partial correlation between the changes after training in anthropometric, cardiometabolic and strength parameters were performed. Statistical significance for all the analyses was defined at $p < 0.05$. SPSS (SPSS 23.0.0.0; SPSS Inc., Chicago, IL, USA) was used for all the statistical calculations.

3. Results

3.1. Participants' General Characteristics

The flow chart with a schematic representation of participant allocation is presented in Figure 1. Forty-five participants met the inclusion criteria: 22 women had been randomly assigned to the HIGH group and 23 to the LOW group. Of them, five subjects abandoned during the intervention period and one was excluded from analysis to prevent outlier bias. Finally, 39 participants were included in the analysis.

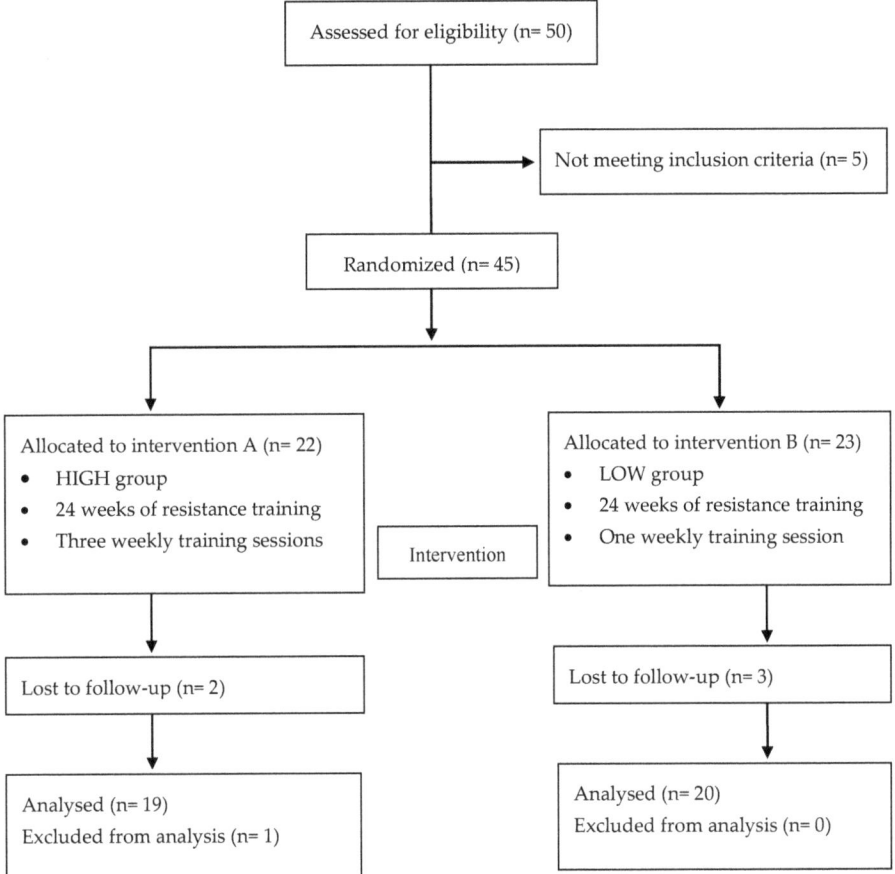

Figure 1. Flow chart.

No significant differences in age, weight, height and BMI were found between the two groups before the intervention period (Table 1).

Table 1. General characteristics of the participants before the intervention period.

Variable		HIGH (n = 22)	LOW (n = 23)	p
Age (years)	a	55.51 ± 9.16	57.50 ± 8.44	0.46
	b	40–69	40–68	
Weight (kg)	a	97.43 ± 17.41	88.76 ± 16.00	0.10
	b	73.50–137.10	73.20–139.30	
Height (cm)	a	158.51 ± 6.12	158.05 ± 6.60	0.81
	b	146.80–170.70	146.00–168.90	
BMI (kg/m^2)	a	38.70 ± 6.18	35.58 ± 6.35	0.11
	b	28.10–52.10	27.50–51.00	

Note: A = mean ± SD, b = range.

3.2. Anthropometry

There was a significant group by time interaction for weight, BMI, WC and the percentage of fat mass (%FM) with an 8.7%, 8.7%, 9.0% and 9.8% decrease in the HIGH group and with a 4.9%, 4.9%, 4.7% and 5.3% decrease in LOW group (Table 2), respectively. After adjusting for age, weight loss, and menopausal status as covariates, the group by time interaction remained significant for weight ($F = 4.15$, $p = 0.049$, statistical power = 0.51), WC ($F = 8.02$, $p = 0.007$, statistical power = 0.78) and %FM ($F = 7.79$, $p = 0.008$, statistical power = 0.77). Post hoc analysis revealed that in both groups all the anthropometric values significantly decreased from before to after the intervention period.

Table 2. Participant characteristics before and after the 24 weeks of intervention.

Variable	HIGH (n = 19)		LOW (n = 20)		ES	Interaction p-Value	SP
	Before	After	Before	After			
Anthropometry							
Weight (kg)	97.43 ± 17.41	88.73 ± 18.52 *	88.76 ± 16.00	84.02 ± 13.20 *	−0.31	<0.01	0.80
BMI (kg/m²)	38.70 ± 6.18	35.25 ± 6.85 *	35.58 ± 6.35	33.66 ± 5.05 *	−0.19	<0.01	0.77
WC (cm)	110.31 ± 13.68	100.49 ± 14.66 *	106.69 ± 12.26	101.46 ± 11.24 *	−0.41	<0.01	0.89
FM (%)	40.17 ± 3.29	36.26 ± 3.73 *	39.36 ± 3.36	37.24 ± 3.70 *	−5.60	<0.01	0.94
Blood pressure							
SBP (mmHg)	130.48 ±13.77	125.24 ± 17.78	127.62 ± 11.46	121.43 ± 25.93	0.04	0.89	0.05
DBP (mmHg)	81.43 ± 9.10	77.57 ± 9.66	78.81 ± 6.69	78.33 ± 10.16	0.35	0.26	0.19
Lipid profile							
TC (mg/dl)	204.50 ± 49.16	196.14 ± 44.08 *	209.85 ± 32.42	202.36 ± 27.87	−0.05	0.87	0.05
TG (mg/dl)	143.35 ± 52.90	120.18 ± 50.28 *	138.54 ± 54.25	127.69 ± 50.44 *	−0.31	0.30	0.17
HDL-C (mg/dl)	54.30 ± 15.16	59.43 ± 16.24 *	53.04 ± 13.74	54.35 ± 13.96 *	0.58	0.06	0.45
LDL-C (mg/dl)	133.58 ± 27.76	121.29 ± 25.00 *	122.98 ± 41.62	120.33 ± 48.75	−0.60	0.05	0.58
Insulin resistance							
HbA1c (%)	6.05 ± 0.65	5.68 ± 0.67 *	6.56 ± 1.36	6.31 ± 1.22 *	−0.39	0.20	0.23
Glucose (mg/dl)	97.48 ± 13.77	88.82 ± 12.89 *	94.98 ± 7.83	92.43 ± 7.54 *	−1.33	<0.01	0.98
Insulin (u/l)	13.07 ± 2.61	11.01 ± 2.90 *	11.63 ± 2.85	10.79 ± 2.71 *	−0.76	0.01	0.68
HOMA$_{IR}$	3.12 ± 0.68	2.40 ± 0.67 *	2.72 ± 0.69	2.45 ± 0.58 *	−1.07	<0.01	0.92
Strength							
DHS (kg)	22.76 ± 4.92	27.04 ± 5.29 *	24.50 ± 5.66	25.45 ± 5.77	1.34	<0.01	0.99
AHS (kg)	42.81 ± 9.39	50.35 ± 9.13 *	46.88 ± 11.18	48.83 ± 11.71	1.36	<0.01	0.99
RHS (kg)	1.12 ± 0.27	1.47 ± 0.36 *	1.34 ± 0.36	1.47 ± 0.39 *	1.53	<0.01	0.98

Note: Data are expressed as the mean and standard deviation. * $p < 0.05$ vs. before, BMI: body mass index, WC: waist circumference, FM: fat mass, SBP: systolic blood pressure, DBP: diastolic blood pressure, TC: total cholesterol, TG: triacylglycerol, LDL-C: low-density lipoprotein cholesterol, HbA1c: glycated hemoglobin, HOMA$_{IR}$: homeostasis model assessment for insulin resistance, DHS: dominant handgrip strength, AHS: Absolute handgrip strength, RHS: relative handgrip strength, SP: statistical power.

Figure 2 shows changes in the weight status categories among the participants after 24 weeks. In the HIGH group, 11 women reached a lower weight status category than at the beginning of the study ($p = 0.001$), while only seven achieved this in the LOW group ($p = 0.01$).

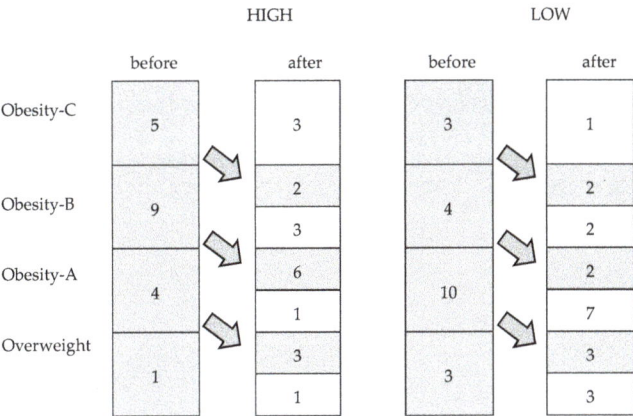

Figure 2. Changes in the weight status categories among the participants after the intervention period.

3.3. Cardiometabolic Risk Factors

A significant group by time interaction was found for plasma glucose, insulin and HOMA$_{IR}$ (Table 2). After adjusting for age, weight loss and menopausal status as covariates, the group by time interaction remained significant for plasma glucose (F = 19.54, $p < 0.001$, statistical power = 0.99), insulin (F = 5.43, $p = 0.025$, statistical power = 0.62), and HOMA$_{IR}$ (F = 10.83, $p = 0.002$, statistical power = 0.89). Post hoc analysis showed that, after the intervention period, the participants significantly reduced their fasting plasma glucose of 8.7% and 2.6%, insulin of 16.0% and 6.5% and HOMA$_{IR}$ of 23% and 8.9% in the HIGH and LOW group, respectively. HbA1c, TC, TG and LDL cholesterol were significantly decreased, and the HDL cholesterol was increased in the HIGH group after the intervention period. HbA1c, TG and HDL cholesterol were similarly changed in the LOW group ($p < 0.05$). The systolic and diastolic blood pressure were not significantly changed in both groups after the 24 week intervention program.

3.4. Handgrip Strength

A significant group by time interaction was also found for the DHS, AHS and RHS (Table 2). After controlling for age, weight loss, and menopausal status as covariates, the group by time interaction was significant for the DHS (F = 15.09, $p < 0.001$, statistical power = 0.96), AHS (F = 15.57, $p < 0.001$, statistical power = 0.97), and the RHS (F = 23.67, $p < 0.001$, statistical power = 0.99). In the HIGH group, participants increased the strength values by 19.8%, 18.7% and 30.1% for the DHS, AHS and RHS, respectively, while for the same parameters in the LOW group the increments were 4.6%, 4.7% and 10.2%, respectively. Post hoc analyses revealed that in the HIGH group, the participants increased their DHS, AHS and RHS after the intervention ($p < 0.05$). On the contrary, the LOW group changed significantly only in RHS.

3.5. Correlations

The matrix of correlations between the percent variations after the Lifestyle program (Δ) in anthropometric parameters, cardiometabolic risk factors and strength values is presented in Table 3. After adjusting for age, weight loss, and menopausal status as covariates, the association remained significant between the weight and WC (r = 0.425, $p = 0.006$), %FM (r = 0.418, $p = 0.007$) glucose (r = 0.374, $p = 0.017$), and RHS (r = −0.422, $p = 0.007$). Other associations were shown between WC and %FM (r = 0.315, $p = 0.048$), HDL cholesterol (r = −0.387, $p = 0.014$), LDL cholesterol (r = 0.356, $p = 0.024$), glucose (r = 0.369, $p = 0.019$), insulin (r = 0.347, $p = 0.028$), HOMA$_{IR}$ (r = 0.407, $p = 0.009$) and RHS (r = −0.392, $p = 0.012$), and between %FM and glucose (r = 0.495, $p = 0.001$), insulin (r = 0.380, p

= 0.015), HOMA$_{IR}$ (r = 0.490, p = 0.001) AHS (r = −0.364, p = 0.021) and RHS (r = −0.513, p < 0.001). Changes in LDL cholesterol were associated with variations in HDL cholesterol (r = −0.357, p = 0.024) and in HbA1c (r = 0.327, p = 0.040). Significantly correlations were also found among the glucose and HOMA$_{IR}$ (r = 0.569, p < 0.001), AHR (r = −0.349, p = 0.027) and RHS (r = −0.480, p = 0.002), and between AHS and HbA1c (p = 0.039), insulin (r = −0.365, p = 0.021), HOMA$_{IR}$ (r = −0.426, p = 0.006), DHS (r = 0.778, p < 0.001) and RHS (r = 0.902, p < 0.001). HOMA$_{IR}$ was also correlated with insulin (r = 0.948, p < 0.001) and RHS (r = −0.500, p = 0.001).

Table 3. Matrix of the correlations between the percentage variations of the variables after training.

	BMI	WC	FM	HDL-C	LDL-C	HbA1c	GLU	INS	HOMA$_{IR}$	AHS	RHS
Weight	1.00 †	0.54 †	0.39 *	−0.24	0.20	0.68	0.47 †	0.29	0.35 *	−0.07	−0.45 *
BMI		1.00	0.53 †	0.38 *	−0.24	0.20	0.06	0.47 †	0.29	0.35 *	−0.06	−0.45 *
WC	-		1.00	0.29	−0.41 *	0.42 *	0.25	0.40 *	0.30 *	0.36 *	−0.21	−0.38 *
FM	-	-		1.00	−0.08	0.36 *	0.24	0.53 †	0.45 *	0.47 †	−0.39 *	−0.47 †
HDL-C	-	-	-		1.00	−0.32 *	−0.01	−0.28	−0.09	−0.16	0.10	0.18
LDL-C	-	-	-	-		1.00	0.40 *	0.21	0.20	0.23	−0.23	−0.27
HbA1c	-	-	-	-	-		1.00	0.07	−0.05	−0.07	−0.32 *	−0.29
GLU	-	-	-	-	-	-		1.00	0.41 *	0.60 †	−0.31 *	−0.47 †
INS	-	-	-	-	-	-	-		1.00	0.95 †	−0.36 *	−0.42 *
HOMA$_{IR}$	-	-	-	-	-	-	-	-		1.00	−0.40 *	−0.47 †
AHS	-	-	-	-	-	-	-	-	-		1.00	0.88 †

Note: * p < 0.05, † p < 0.001, GLU: glucose, INS: insulin.

4. Discussion

We found that 24 weeks of resistance training improved health in overweight and obese participants. Our resistance training program led to weight loss and a reduced BMI, improved insulin resistance and fat mass profile, and increased relative strength in participants. Aronne and Isoldi [41] suggested that changes in anthropometric and cardiometabolic risk factors are essential to improve obese health outcomes. Although some studies reported a statistically insignificant trend or no change in fat mass after a resistance training program [42,43], our study is in line with the findings of other authors who reported beneficial changes in body composition [44], fat mass and fat-free mass [45,46], muscle volume [47], physical function [48], BMI [49], and body weight [50]. According to Kraemer and Ratamess [35], the foremost principles of resistance training progression are progressive overload, specificity, and variation. We assessed these altering exercise intensity and training volume. However, one limitation may be that we never changed the exercise selection and rest over time.

We also hypothesized that the highest training frequency would have provided more positive improvements in body composition, cardiometabolic risk factors, and handgrip strength. No prior evidence was available on the differences in training frequencies in obese and overweight people. The American College of Sports Medicine [51] recommended that novice individuals should do full body resistance exercise 2–3 days per week. Our results agreed with it and showed that a higher frequency better affects obese and overweight health in women. The most important differences between the two groups relate to some of the lipid profile parameters, such as total cholesterol, LDL cholesterol, and handgrip strength. In the group that followed the resistance training program three times a week, these parameters increased significantly, unlike the group that trained once per week.

Another important result of our study was that a 24 week exercise program elicited a positive effect on metabolic syndrome risk factors such as HbA1c, HOMA$_{IR}$ and lipid profile. A review from Lee and colleagues [19] showed that resistance exercise improved insulin resistance and lipid profile in younger obese, but the best outcomes appeared with resistance combined with aerobic exercise. In addition, Brown and associates [52] showed that a single bout of resistance exercise positively affected the glucose and insulin level during 18–24 h post exercise. However, more evidence is needed.

No significant changes in blood pressure values were measured after the intervention in both groups, though they tended towards improvements. Similar results were found by Sigal and colleagues [53], who could not find reductions in blood pressure values after 22 weeks in the participants of a resistance training program, and not even in those who practiced an aerobic training program. A limitation in our results may be due to the experimental designs that did not include diet with a caloric restriction program. Several authors found that dietary patterns combined with exercise improved obese health [54,55].

Our view is that high-frequency training is crucial in the development of strength, which also plays an important role in cardiovascular health. On this point, Lee et al. [56] reported that handgrip strength is correlated with cardiometabolic risk factors including blood pressure, triglyceride, HDL cholesterol, HbA1c, and fasting glucose. In line with that, our results highlighted significant correlations between handgrip strength and HbA1c, plasma glucose, plasma insulin and $HOMA_{IR}$, indicating that strength development may have played a role in improving insulin resistance and cardiometabolic risk factor. Moreover, the observed increase in the handgrip strength concomitant with an improved insulin resistance sensitivity after training constituted an essential element for cardiovascular health.

Other limitations of our study included: (a) we did not consider a control group to monitor the differences of the changes in the evaluated parameters between those who practice a controlled exercise and those who do not; (b) only women were included in this experimental design, therefore our findings may not be applicable on a male sample; (c) we were not able to monitor physical activity levels outside of the study environment and to track dietary intake throughout the study, though individuals were asked to maintain their usual lifestyle habits.

Further evidence on the subject could be collected, contributing to this particular field of research and supporting the effort of clinicians working with physical exercise for obese or overweight people. The literature is abundant with resistance training studies, but very little is known regarding the effects of different frequencies of weekly training. As demonstrated by our results, resistance exercise and its weekly training frequency causes different effects on body composition, cardiometabolic risk factors and in particular on strength development. In fact, although both groups had an improvement trend after 24 weeks of intervention, the major effects on the examined parameters were measured in the group that performed the training program at a higher weekly frequency.

5. Conclusions

Resistance training is effective to induce improvement in body composition and cardiometabolic risk factors, but the development of handgrip strength can only be achieved with a high training frequency. This study shows that a high training frequency gave greater benefits for weight loss, cardiometabolic risk factor improvement, and handgrip strength, than a training program with a session of once a week.

Author Contributions: Conceptualization, F.C., G.G. and S.T.; data curation, F.S. and S.T.; formal analysis, F.C., G.G. and M.M.; investigation, F.C. and M.M.; methodology, P.M.L. and G.G.; project administration, P.M.L.; resources, P.M.L. and F.S.; software, P.M.; supervision, S.T.; validation, F.C.; visualization, P.M.L. and F.S.; writing—original draft, F.C.; writing—review and editing, F.C., G.G. and M.M. All authors have read and agreed to the published version of the manuscript.

Funding: This research received no external funding.

Acknowledgments: The authors are grateful to all the participants who took part in this study and to the research assistants who contributed to the collection of data and to the supervision of the Exercise program.

Conflicts of Interest: The authors declare no conflict of interest.

References

1. World Health Organization. Obesity. Available online: https://www.who.int/health-topics/obesity#tab=tab_1 (accessed on 12 May 2020).
2. National Institutes of Health. Clinical Guidelines on the Identification, Evaluation, and Treatment of Overweight and Obesity in Adults—The Evidence Report. National Institutes of Health. *Obes. Res.* **1998**, *6*, 51S–209S.

3. Hales, C.M.; Carroll, M.D.; Fryar, C.D.; Ogden, C.L. Prevalence of obesity and severe obesity among adults: United States, 2017–2018. In *NCHS Data Brief*; No. 360; National Center for Health Statistics: Hyattsville, MD, USA, 2020.
4. National Health Statistic. Health Survey of England 2017. Overweight and Obesity in Adults and Children. Available online: https://digital.nhs.uk/data-and-information/publications/statistical/health-survey-for-england/2017 (accessed on 10 May 2020).
5. Farrag, N.S.; Cheskin, L.J.; Farag, M.K. A systematic review of childhood obesity in the Middle East and North Africa (MENA) region: Health impact and management. *Adv. Ped. Res.* **2017**, *4*, 6.
6. NCD Risk Factor Collaboration (NCD-RisC). Worldwide trends in body-mass index, underweight, overweight, and obesity from 1975 to 2016: A pooled analysis of 2416 population-based measurement studies in 128·9 million children, adolescents, and adults. *Lancet* **2017**, *390*, 2627–2642. [CrossRef]
7. Porter Starr, K.N.; McDonald, S.R.; Bales, C.W. Obesity and physical frailty in older adults: A scoping review of lifestyle intervention trials. *J. Am. Med. Direct. Assoc.* **2014**, *15*, 240–250. [CrossRef] [PubMed]
8. Huck, C.J. Effects of supervised resistance training on fitness and functional strength in patients succeeding bariatric surgery. *J. Strength Cond. Res.* **2015**, *29*, 589–595. [CrossRef]
9. Toselli, S.; Gualdi-Russo, E.; Campa, F. Ethnic differences in body image perception in patients with type 2 diabetes. *J. Hum. Nutr. Diet.* **2019**, *32*, 356–371. [CrossRef]
10. Toselli, S.; Gualdi-Russo, E.; Mazzuca, P.; Campa, F. Ethnic differences in body composition, sociodemographic characteristics and lifestyle in people with type 2 diabetes mellitus living in Italy. *Endocrine* **2019**, *65*, 558–568. [CrossRef]
11. Ma, C.; Avenell, A.; Bolland, M.; Hudson, J.; Stewart, F.; Robertson, C.; Sharma, P.; Fraser, C.; MacLennan, G. Effects of weight loss interventions for adults who are obese on mortality, cardiovascular disease, and cancer: Systematic review and meta-analysis. *BMJ (Clin. Res. Ed.)* **2017**, *359*, j4849. [CrossRef]
12. Scott, D.; Harrison, C.L.; Hutchison, S.; de Courten, B.; Stepto, N.K. Exploring factors related to changes in body composition, insulin sensitivity and aerobic capacity in response to a 12-week exercise intervention in overweight and obese women with and without polycystic ovary syndrome. *PLoS ONE* **2017**, *12*, e0182412. [CrossRef]
13. National Heart, Lung, and Blood Institute. Managing Overweight and Obesity in Adults: Systematic Evidence Review from the Obesity Expert Panel. Available online: https://www.nhlbi.nih.gov/sites/default/files/media/docs/obesity-evidence-review.pdf (accessed on 3 May 2020).
14. Theodorakopoulos, C.; Jones, J.; Bannerman, E.; Greig, C.A. Effectiveness of nutritional and exercise interventions to improve body composition and muscle strength or function in sarcopenic obese older adults: A systematic review. *Nutr. Res.* **2017**, *43*, 3–15. [CrossRef]
15. Brown, J.D.; Buscemi, J.; Milsom, V.; Malcolm, R.; O'Neil, P.M. Effects on cardiovascular risk factors of weight losses limited to 5–10. *Transl. Behav. Med.* **2016**, *6*, 339–346. [CrossRef] [PubMed]
16. National Institute for Clinical Excellence (NICE). *Weight Management: Lifestyle Services for Overweight or Obese Adults (NICE guidance PH53)*; National Institute for Health and Care Excellence: London, UK, 2014. Available online: https://www.nice.org.uk/guidance/ph53/chapter/Introduction-scope-and-purpose-of-this-guidance (accessed on 8 May 2020).
17. Etemad, Z.; Moradiani, H.; Aziz-Beigi, K. Adiponectin is associated with inflammatory markers and insulin resistance following moderate-intensity circuit weight training in healthy overweight and obese men. *Med. Sport* **2015**, *68*, 627–638.
18. Rajagopalan, P.; Dixit, S.; Alahmari, K.; Devenesan, C.S.; Rengaramanujam, K.; Zaman, G.S.; Ali Asiri, H.; Chandramoorthy, C.H. Resistance training influences Adipokines and various biochemical factors altering the risk of metabolic syndrome in young male obese students. *Med. Sport* **2018**, *71*, 561–578.
19. Lee, S.; Kim, Y.; Kuk, J.L. What Is the Role of Resistance Exercise in Improving the Cardiometabolic Health of Adolescents with Obesity? *J. Obes. Metab. Syndr.* **2019**, *28*, 76–91. [CrossRef] [PubMed]
20. Christiansen, T.; Paulsen, S.K.; Bruun, J.M.; Pedersen, S.B.; Richelsen, B. Exercise training versus diet-induced weight-loss on metabolic risk factors and inflammatory markers in obese subjects: A 12-week randomized intervention study. American journal of physiology. *Endoc. Met.* **2010**, *298*, E824–E831. [CrossRef]
21. Straight, C.R.; Dorfman, L.R.; Cottell, K.E.; Krol, J.M.; Lofgren, I.E.; Delmonico, M.J. Effects of resistance training and dietary changes on physical function and body composition in overweight and obese older adults. *J. Phys. Act. Health* **2012**, *9*, 875–883. [CrossRef]

22. Toselli, S.; Campa, F.; Spiga, F.; Grigoletto, A.; Simonelli, I.; Gualdi-Russo, E. The association between body composition and quality of life among elderly Italians. *Endocrine* **2020**, *68*, 279–286. [CrossRef]
23. Al-Shreef, F.M.; Al-Jiffri, O.H.; Abd El-Kader, S.M. Bone metabolism and hand grip strength response to aerobic versus resistance exercise training in non-insulin dependent diabetic patients. *Afr. Health Sci.* **2015**, *15*, 896–901. [CrossRef]
24. Fazelifar, S.; Ebrahim, K.; Sarkisian, V. Effect of exercise training and detraining on serum leptin levels in obese young boys. *Med. Sport* **2013**, *66*, 325–337.
25. Campa, F.; Silva, A.M.; Toselli, S. Changes in Phase Angle and Handgrip Strength Induced by Suspension Training in Older Women. *Int. J. Sports Med.* **2018**, *39*, 442–449. [CrossRef] [PubMed]
26. Kim, H.J.; Lee, H.J.; So, B.; Son, J.S.; Yoon, D.; Song, W. Effect of aerobic training and resistance training on circulating irisin level and their association with change of body composition in overweight/obese adults: A pilot study. *Physiol. Res.* **2016**, *65*, 271–279. [CrossRef] [PubMed]
27. Filho, J.C.; Gobbi, L.T.; Gurjão, A.L.; Gonçalves, R.; Prado, A.K.; Gobbi, S. Effect of different rest intervals, between sets, on muscle performance during leg press exercise, in trained older women. *J. Sports Sci. Med.* **2013**, *12*, 138–143. [PubMed]
28. Cavalcante, E.F.; Ribeiro, A.S.; do Nascimento, M.A.; Silva, A.M.; Tomeleri, C.M.; Nabuco, H.; Pina, F.; Mayhew, J.L.; Da Silva-Grigoletto, M.E.; da Silva, D.; et al. Effects of Different Resistance Training Frequencies on Fat in Overweight/Obese Older Women. *Int. J. Sports Med.* **2018**, *12*, 527–534. [CrossRef] [PubMed]
29. Harris, C.; DeBeliso, M.A.; Spitzer-Gibson, T.A.; Adams, K.J. The effect of resistance-training intensity on strength-gain response in the older adult. *J. Strength Cond. Res.* **2004**, *18*, 833–838.
30. Sayers, S.P.; Gibson, K. Effects of high-speed power training on muscle performance and braking speed in older adults. *J. Aging Res.* **2012**, *2012*, 426278. [CrossRef]
31. Murlasits, Z.; Reed, J.; Wells, K. Effect of resistance training frequency on physiological adaptations in older adults. *J. Exer. Sci. Fit.* **2012**, *10*, 28–32. [CrossRef]
32. Schulz, K.F.; Altman, D.G.; Moher, D.; CONSORT Group. CONSORT 2010 Statement: Updated guidelines for reporting parallel group randomised trials. *J. Clin. Epidem.* **2010**, *63*, 834–840. [CrossRef]
33. Toselli, S.; Badicu, G.; Bragonzoni, L.; Spiga, F.; Mazzuca, P.; Campa, F. Comparison of the Effect of Different Resistance Training Frequencies on Phase Angle and Handgrip Strength in Obese Women: A Randomized Controlled Trial. *IJERPH* **2020**, *17*, 1163. [CrossRef]
34. Ehrman, K.J.; Gordon, M.P.; Visich, S.P.; Keteyian, J.S. *Clinical Exercise Physiology*, 4th ed.; Human Kinetics Books: Champaign, IL, USA, 2019; pp. 129–136.
35. Kraemer, W.J.; Ratamess, N.A. Fundamentals of resistance training: Progression and exercise prescription. *Med. Sci. Sports Exerc.* **2004**, *36*, 674–688. [CrossRef]
36. Lohman, T.G.; Roche, A.F.; Martorell, R. *Anthropometric Standardization Reference Manual*; Human Kinetics Books: Champaign, IL, USA, 1998.
37. Durnin, J.V.; Womersley, J. Body fat assessed from total body density and its estimation from skinfold thickness: Measurements on 481 men and women aged from 16 to 72 years. *Brit. J. Nutr.* **1974**, *32*, 77–97. [CrossRef]
38. Siri, W.E. Body composition from fluid spaces and density: Analyses of methods. In *Techniques for Measuring Body Composition*; The National Academies National Research Council: Washington, DC, USA, 1961; pp. 223–244.
39. Aruga, M.; Tokita, Y.; Nakajima, K.; Kamachi, K.; Tanaka, A. The effect of combined diet and exercise intervention on body weight and the serum GPIHBP1 concentration in overweight/obese middle-aged women. *Clin. Chim. Acta Int. J. Clin. Chem.* **2017**, *475*, 109–115. [CrossRef] [PubMed]
40. Choquette, S.; Bouchard, D.R.; Doyon, C.Y.; Sénéchal, M.; Brochu, M.; Dionne, I.J. Relative strength as a determinant of mobility in elders 67–84 years of age. a nuage study: Nutrition as a determinant of successful aging. *J. Nutr. Health Aging* **2010**, *14*, 190–195. [CrossRef] [PubMed]
41. Aronne, L.J.; Isoldi, K.K. Overweight and obesity: Key components of cardiometabolic risk. *Clin. Cornerstone* **2007**, *8*, 29–37. [CrossRef]
42. Dos Santos, L.; Cyrino, E.S.; Antunes, M.; Santos, D.A.; Sardinha, L.B. Changes in phase angle and body composition induced by resistance training in older women. *Europ. J. Clin. Nutr.* **2016**, *70*, 1408–1413. [CrossRef] [PubMed]

43. Hansen, D.; Dendale, P.; Berger, J.; van Loon, L.J.; Meeusen, R. The effects of exercise training on fat-mass loss in obese patients during energy intake restriction. *Sports Med.* **2007**, *37*, 31–46. [CrossRef] [PubMed]
44. Beavers, K.M.; Ambrosius, W.T.; Rejeski, W.J.; Burdette, J.H.; Walkup, M.P.; Sheedy, J.L.; Nesbit, B.A.; Gaukstern, J.E.; Nicklas, B.J.; Marsh, A.P. Effect of Exercise Type During Intentional Weight Loss on Body Composition in Older Adults with Obesity. *Obesity* **2017**, *25*, 1823–1829. [CrossRef] [PubMed]
45. Willis, L.H.; Slentz, C.A.; Bateman, L.A.; Shields, A.T.; Piner, L.W.; Bales, C.W.; Houmard, J.A.; Kraus, W.E. Effects of aerobic and/or resistance training on body mass and fat mass in overweight or obese adults. *J. Appl. Physiol.* **2012**, *113*, 1831–1837. [CrossRef] [PubMed]
46. Alberga, A.S.; Farnesi, B.C.; Lafleche, A.; Legault, L.; Komorowski, J. The effects of resistance exercise training on body composition and strength in obese prepubertal children. *Physic. Sportsmed.* **2013**, *41*, 103–109. [CrossRef]
47. Keating, S.E.; Hackett, D.A.; Parker, H.M.; Way, K.L.; O'Connor, H.T.; Sainsbury, A.; Baker, M.K.; Chuter, V.H.; Caterson, I.D.; George, J.; et al. Effect of resistance training on liver fat and visceral adiposity in adults with obesity: A randomized controlled trial. *Hepatol. Res. Off. J. Jpn. Soc. Hepatol.* **2017**, *47*, 622–631. [CrossRef]
48. Liao, C.D.; Tsauo, J.Y.; Huang, S.W.; Ku, J.W.; Hsiao, D.J.; Liou, T.H. Effects of elastic band exercise on lean mass and physical capacity in older women with sarcopenic obesity: A randomized controlled trial. *Scient. Rep.* **2018**, *8*, 2317. [CrossRef]
49. Freitas, P.D.; Silva, A.G.; Ferreira, P.G.; DA Silva, A.; Salge, J.M.; Carvalho-Pinto, R.M.; Cukier, A.; Brito, C.M.; Mancini, M.C.; Carvalho, C. Exercise Improves Physical Activity and Comorbidities in Obese Adults with Asthma. *Med. Sci. Sports Exerc.* **2018**, *50*, 1367–1376. [CrossRef] [PubMed]
50. Villareal, D.T.; Aguirre, L.; Gurney, A.B.; Waters, D.L.; Sinacore, D.R.; Colombo, E.; Armamento-Villareal, R.; Qualls, C. Aerobic or resistance exercise, or both, in dieting obese older adults. *N. Engl. J. Med.* **2017**, *376*, 1943–1955. [CrossRef] [PubMed]
51. American College of Sports Medicine. American College of Sports Medicine position stand. Progression models in resistance training for healthy adults. *Med. Sci. Sports Exerc.* **2009**, *41*, 687–708. [CrossRef]
52. Brown, E.C.; Franklin, B.A.; Regensteiner, J.G.; Stewart, K.J. Effects of single bout resistance exercise on glucose levels, insulin action, and cardiovascular risk in type 2 diabetes: A narrative review. *J. Diab. Complic.* **2020**, *34*, 107610. [CrossRef] [PubMed]
53. Fock, K.M.; Khoo, J. Diet and exercise in management of obesity and overweight. *J. Gastroent. Hepatol.* **2013**, *28*, 59–63. [CrossRef]
54. Franz, M.J.; VanWormer, J.J.; Crain, A.L.; Boucher, J.L.; Histon, T.; Caplan, W.; Bowman, J.D.; Pronk, N.P. Weight-loss outcomes: A systematic review and meta-analysis of weight-loss clinical trials with a minimum 1-year follow-up. *J. Am. Diet. Assoc.* **2007**, *107*, 1755–1767. [CrossRef]
55. Sigal, R.J.; Kenny, G.P.; Boulé, N.G.; Wells, G.A.; Prud'homme, D.; Fortier, M.; Reid, R.D.; Tulloch, H.; Coyle, D.; Phillips, P.; et al. Effects of aerobic training, resistance training, or both on glycemic control in type 2 diabetes: A randomized trial. *Ann. Int. Med.* **2007**, *147*, 357–369. [CrossRef]
56. Lee, W.J.; Peng, L.N.; Chiou, S.T.; Chen, L.K. Relative Handgrip Strength Is a Simple Indicator of Cardiometabolic Risk among Middle-Aged and Older People: A Nationwide Population-Based Study in Taiwan. *PLoS ONE* **2016**, *11*, e0160876. [CrossRef]

© 2020 by the authors. Licensee MDPI, Basel, Switzerland. This article is an open access article distributed under the terms and conditions of the Creative Commons Attribution (CC BY) license (http://creativecommons.org/licenses/by/4.0/).

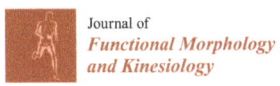

Article

Associations between Activity Pacing, Fatigue, and Physical Activity in Adults with Multiple Sclerosis: A Cross Sectional Study

Ulric S. Abonie [1,2], **Femke Hoekstra** [3,4], **Bregje L. Seves** [3], **Lucas H. V. van der Woude** [3,4], **Rienk Dekker** [4] **and Florentina J. Hettinga** [5,*]

1. Department of Physiotherapy and Rehabilitation Sciences, University of Health and Allied Sciences, Ho PMB 31 Volta Region, Ghana; uabonie@uhas.edu.gh
2. School of Sport, Rehabilitation and Exercise Science, University of Essex, Colchester CO4 3SQ, Essex, UK
3. Center for Human Movement Sciences, University Medical Center Groningen, University of Groningen, PO Box 72, 9700 AB Groningen, The Netherlands; fhoekstra@mail.ubc.ca (F.H.); b.l.seves@umcg.nl (B.L.S.); l.h.v.van.der.woude@umcg.nl (L.H.V.v.d.W.)
4. Department of Rehabilitation, University Medical Center Groningen, University of Groningen, PO Box 72, 9700 AB Groningen, The Netherlands; r.dekker01@umcg.nl
5. Department of Sport, Exercise and Rehabilitation, Northumbria University, Newcastle upon Tyne NE1 8SB, UK
* Correspondence: florentina.hettinga@northumbria.ac.uk; Tel.: +44-77-648-853-76

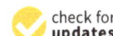

Received: 13 April 2020; Accepted: 9 June 2020; Published: 15 June 2020

Abstract: Fatigue is common in people with multiple sclerosis (MS). Activity pacing is a behavioral way to cope with fatigue and limited energy resources. However, little is known about how people with MS naturally pace activities to manage their fatigue and optimize daily activities. This study explored how activity pacing relates to fatigue and physical activity in people with MS. Participants were 80 individuals (60 females, 20 males) with a diagnosis of MS. The participants filled in questionnaires on their activity pacing, fatigue, physical activity, and health-related quality of life, 3–6 weeks before discharge from rehabilitation. The relationships between the variables were examined using hierarchical regression. After controlling for demographics, health-related quality of life, and perceived risk of overactivity, no associations were found between activity pacing and fatigue ($\beta = 0.20$; t = 1.43, $p = 0.16$) or between activity pacing and physical activity ($\beta = -0.24$; t = −1.61, $p = 0.12$). The lack of significant associations between activity pacing and fatigue or physical activity suggests that without interventions, there appears to be no clear strategy amongst people with MS to manage fatigue and improve physical activity. People with MS may benefit from interventions to manage fatigue and optimize engagement in physical activity.

Keywords: activity pacing; multiple sclerosis; perceived risk of overactivity; perceived fatigue; health-related quality of life; rehabilitation

---

1. Introduction

Symptoms of fatigue are among the most frequently reported and strongest predictors of functional disability in people with multiple sclerosis (MS) [1–3]. The experience of fatigue and perceived fatigability (changes in the sensations that regulates effort and endurance) draws behavioral adaptations, such as limiting the engagement in activities resulting in underactivity, or a lifestyle characterized by periods of overactivity followed by long extensive rest periods [4–7]. However, both underactivity and overactivity are linked with disability [8].

Despite growing efforts to manage fatigue through exercise interventions in people with MS, studies investigating the effect of exercise interventions report a high number of dropouts, and identified that participants struggle to continue engaging in physical activity post-intervention [9,10]. This warrants the need to explore ways to enable long-term adoption of a physically active lifestyle.

Activity pacing is a self-management strategy that can help alter often-occurring inefficient activity patterns (underactivity and overactivity) and stimulate long-term engagement in an active lifestyle [11]. It involves dividing one's daily activities into smaller, manageable pieces to manage fatigue, and to maintain a steady activity pace, whilst reducing relapses [12,13]. However, current literature on how people naturally pace activities in daily life is limited and inconclusive [11–16]; some studies show that activity pacing is associated with higher levels of fatigue and lower physical activity [16,17], while others show the opposite or no association [8,18], and no clear strategies are available in rehabilitation treatment to optimize activity pacing to improve engagement in physical activity [14]. Similarly, quality of life has been proposed to impact activity pacing [8].

It is notable that most of the above studies aimed to explore issues in a range of chronic disabling conditions and did not focus on MS specifically. Thus while findings from these studies [8,13–18] contribute to our understanding of activity pacing, their broader focus with regards to multiple health behaviors and mixed populations may have resulted in failure to elicit key issues specific to engagement in physical activity for people with MS. Currently no study has explored people with MS in a natural approach to activity pacing, and its relations to fatigue and physical activity.

Understanding these associations can help guide and tailor rehabilitation treatment efforts for people with MS and promote an active lifestyle in this population. The aim of this study was to examine reported engagement in pacing and how it relates to fatigue and physical activity in people with MS just before discharge from rehabilitation, controlling for demographics, health-related quality of life, and perceived risk of overactivity. Based on the expectation that activity pacing would be an adaptive strategy to manage fatigue and optimize daily activities [14,17], we hypothesized that reported engagement in pacing would be associated with a decrease in fatigue and an increase in physical activity.

2. Materials and Methods

2.1. Design

This study was part of a multicenter longitudinal study (Rehabilitation, Sports, and Active lifestyle; ReSpAct) to evaluate the nationwide implementation of an active lifestyle program (Rehabilitation, Sports, and Exercise; RSE) among people with a wide range of chronic diseases and/or physical disabilities in Dutch rehabilitation [19,20]. Participants received either inpatient or outpatient rehabilitation at rehabilitation centers and departments of rehabilitation in hospitals because of MS. The current study uses a cross-sectional design based on baseline measurement (3–6 weeks before discharge from rehabilitation) of activity pacing behaviors, fatigue, physical activity, and health-related quality of life of people with MS, selected from the ReSpAct dataset. The study procedures were approved by the ethics committee of the Center for Human Movement Sciences of the University Medical Center Groningen, University of Groningen (reference: ECB/2013.02.28_1) and at participating institutions.

2.2. Participants

Participants were recruited upon referral to the participating rehabilitation institutions across the Netherlands. Potential participants received information on study rationale and procedures, had questions answered, and were checked for the inclusion criteria. Participants were included in this study if they were 18 years and older, had a diagnosis of MS, had received rehabilitation care or treatment based on medicine consultation within one of the participating rehabilitation institutions, and participated in the 'RSE' program. Participants were excluded from the study if they were not able to complete the questionnaires, even with help, or participated in another physical activity stimulation program. Eligible participants who volunteered signed an informed consent form.

2.3. Procedure

Enrolled participants were assessed through a standardized baseline measurement, which consisted of filling out a set of questionnaires on paper or digitally [19,21–23]. As part of the full questionnaire and producer, first, participants indicated which physical activities they perform in the context of the rehabilitation treatment and on their own initiative by filling out an adapted version of the short questionnaire to assess health enhancing physical activity (SQUASH) [21]. Secondly, participants filled out short questionnaires on their perceived engagement in pacing, risk of overactivity, and fatigue [19,22]. Lastly, participants filled out a questionnaire on their health-related quality of life [23].

2.4. Measures

2.4.1. Primary Measures

Fatigue severity was measured using the Fatigue Severity Scale (FSS) [22], a valid and reliable questionnaire to determine the impact of fatigue in people with MS [24]. The participants scored the nine items of the questionnaire on a scale of 1–7 (1, completely disagree; 7 completely agree). Mean fatigue score based on an average of the nine items was used. The mean fatigue score ranges from 1 to 7. A mean FSS score ≥4 was adopted as the cut-off for clinically significant fatigue [25].

Physical activity was assessed using an adapted version of the Short Questionnaire to Assess Health-Enhancing Physical Activity [21]. The questionnaire is a self-reported recall measure to assess daily physical activity based on an average week in the past month. The original questionnaire has demonstrated good test–retest reliability and internal consistency and moderate concurrent validity in ordering participants according to their level of physical activity [21,26,27]. Some minor changes were made to make the SQUASH applicable for people with a chronic disease or physical disability. Specifically, within the domains 'commuting activities', 'leisure-time', and 'sports activities', the items 'wheelchair riding' and 'hand cycling' were added. Also, 'tennis' was modified as '(wheelchair) tennis'. Total minutes of physical activity per week was calculated by multiplying frequency (days/week) and duration (minutes/day) for each activity.

Reported engagement in pacing was assessed with the 'engagement in pacing' subscale of the Activity Pacing and Risk of Overactivity Questionnaire [19]. This questionnaire was developed for use in the ReSpAct study [19]. The engagement in pacing subscale reflected reported engagement in pacing within daily routines and was the primary outcome in the current study. Participants scored the five items of the subscale on a scale of 1–5 (1, never; 2, rarely; 3, sometimes; 4, often; 5, very often). The mean subscale score ranged from 1 to 5, with higher score indicating high engagement in pacing.

Appendix A shows the preliminary validation metrics of the questionnaire. In summary, the sampling adequacy tested with the Kaiser–Myer–Olkin (KMO) and the Bartlett's test of sphericity showed that the questionnaire had a KMO of 0.722, and Bartlett's test was significant ($p < 0.05$), supporting a principal component analysis (PCA). Results of the PCA showed that there were two factors with an Eigen value >1.00, therefore based on the Kaiser's criterion two components were chosen. Factor loadings were used to assign the items to the two components. The two components explained 60.50% of the total variance and there was a negative correlation between the two components of −0.115.

2.4.2. Background Measures and Confounders

Background demographics included age, gender, and body mass index, which was calculated from self-reported body mass and height (body mass (kg)/height^2 (m^2)).

To assess health-related quality of life, the RAND-12-Item Health Survey (RAND-12) [23] was used. RAND-12 assesses seven health domains; general health, physical functioning, role limitations due to physical health problem bodily pain, role limitations due to emotional problems, vitality/mental health, and social functioning. The RAND-12 was scored using the recommended scoring algorithm for calculating general health [28], a composite score of person's health-related quality of life. Scores ranged from 18 to 62. A high score indicated better health-related quality of life. The RAND-12 has been proven to be a valid and reliable measure of health-related quality of life [29].

The 'risk of overactivity' subscale of the Activity Pacing and Risk of Overactivity Questionnaire [19] was used to measure perceived risk of overactivity within daily routines. Participants scored the two items of the subscale on a scale of 1–5 (1, never; 2, rarely; 3, sometimes; 4, often; 5, very often). The mean score ranged from 1 to 5, with higher score indicating high perceived risk of overactivity.

2.5. Data Analysis

Data were analyzed using IBM Statistical Package for the Social Sciences version 23.0 [30]. Based on descriptive statistics and visual inspection of frequency distributions, data were normally distributed. All values were reported using descriptive statistics of means, standard deviations, and interquartile ranges to summarize characteristics of participants. To ensure there was no multicollinearity, bivariate Pearson correlations were conducted to examine basic between-person associations among demographic and study variables, prior to testing the study hypotheses (variables were not highly correlated with each other, $r < 0.8$).

Hierarchical linear regression was used to test the study hypotheses. This statistical approach was optimal for adjustment for confounders, as we wanted to determine whether there were relationships between engagement in pacing and fatigue, and between engagement in pacing and physical activity after controlling for demographics, health-related quality of life, and perceived risk of overactivity.

To examine how engagement in pacing was related to fatigue and physical activity, two hierarchical regression analyses were conducted with fatigue or physical activity as the dependent variable, and engagement in pacing as the independent variable. Age, gender, body mass index, health-related quality of life, and perceived risk of overactivity were confounders.

These demographics and confounders were included in the models based on the fact that they are general demographic variables of interest in studies on physical activity behaviour and fatigue experience, and on known associations with perceived fatigability and physical activity behaviour [18,31]. We chose to analyze our data using these models based on the literature and our expectation that activity pacing may be a positive strategy to manage fatigue and optimize daily activities [14,15].

In both models, at the first step, gender, age, and body mass index were entered. At the second step, health-related quality of life and perceived risk of overactivity were entered, and at the third step engagement in pacing was entered. In both models, the variance inflation factors (VIFs) were examined for multicollinearity.

3. Results

Of the 89 participants included in the study, nine participants had incomplete data and were therefore excluded from the analysis. Characteristics of the sample ($N = 80$) are shown in Table 1. Of the sample, 75% were female ($n = 60$) and the mean age was 44 ± 11 years. The majority of the sample ($n = 73$, 91.3%) were scored as having clinically significant fatigue on the FSS (FSS score > 4). We found that 85.61% ($n = 69$) of the participants lived independently and 33.6% ($n = 69$) had a university education. The sample was, on average, overweight according the World Health Organization standards (body mass index ≥ 25.0 kg/m^2).

Bivariate Pearson correlations (Table 2) showed that the variables were not strongly correlated with each other, providing support for the decision to include them into the primary analyses. Fatigue and health-related quality of life had the highest modest correlation ($r = -0.41$). The next modest correlations were between engagement in pacing and health-related quality of life ($r = -0.27$), and between engagement in pacing and fatigue ($r = 0.27$). These were followed by the correlations between engagement in pacing and physical activity ($r = -0.25$), and between engagement in pacing and age ($r = 0.24$). All other bivariate correlations were of modest magnitude ($r \leq \pm 0.22$).

Table 1. Demographics of Participants ($N = 80$).

Variable	Mean ± SD or N (%)	Interquartile Range *	Scale Range
Age (years)	44.48 ± 10.67	38.00–52.00	22–68
Body mass index (kg/m^2)	27.28 ± 6.91	23.04–32.41	18–53
Number of women (%)	60 (75)		
Living situation (lives alone)	69 (85.61)		
High education level [a]	27 (33.6)		
Engagement in pacing	3.74 ± 0.71	3.30–4.20	1–5
Perceived risk of overactivity	3.73 ± 0.86	3.00–4.50	1–5
Fatigue severity	5.43 ± 1.11	4.78–6.17	1–7
Physical activity (minutes/week)	1585.64 ± 1103.51	780.00–2070.00	
Health-related quality of life	34.35 ± 7.73	28.03–40.26	18–62

* Interquartile range of the 25th percentile and the 75th percentile. [a] Completed university or higher.

Table 2. Bivariate Pearson correlations of all variables in the hierarchical linear regression models.

Variables	2	3	4	5	6	7	8
1. Engagement in pacing	−0.21	0.27 *	−0.25 *	−0.27 *	0.24 *	0.05	−0.20
2. Perceived risk of overactivity		0.19	0.14	−0.16	−0.10	−0.04	0.21
3. Fatigue			−0.14	−0.41 **	0.04	0.04	−0.02
4. Physical activity				−0.02	−0.15	0.08	0.09
5. Health-related quality of life					0.12	−0.05	−0.4
6. Age						−0.22	−0.17
7. Gender							−0.12
8. Body mass index							1

* Correlation is significant at the 0.05 level. ** Correlation is significant at the 0.01 level.

3.1. Primary Analyses

3.1.1. Relationship between Engagement in Pacing and Fatigue

Results of the relationship between engagement in pacing and fatigue, controlling for demographics and confounders (Table 3), showed no association between engagement in pacing and fatigue ($\beta = 0.198$; $t = 1.43$, $p = 0.16$). Among the confounders, health-related quality of life was negatively related to fatigue ($\beta = -0.341$; $t = -2.57$, $p = 0.03$).

Table 3. Hierarchical linear regression model showing the relationship between engagement in pacing and fatigue.

Variable	β	B	SE	df	t	p-Value
Age	0.058	0.006	0.014	3, 55	0.436	0.664
Gender	0.065	0.155	0.302	3, 55	0.515	0.609
Body mass index	−0.011	−0.002	0.021	3, 55	−0.086	0.931
Health-related quality of life	−0.341	−0.049	0.019	2, 53	−2.568	0.013
Perceived risk of overactivity	0.188	0.243	0.167	2, 53	1.454	0.152
Engagement in pacing	0.198	0.307	0.215	1, 52	1.431	0.158

β, Standardized regression coefficients from the complete regression model accounting for all variables; B, unstandardized regression coefficients from the complete regression model accounting for all variables; df, degree of freedom; SE, standard error of B. Note: In this model, fatigue was the dependent variable, engagement in pacing was an independent variable, and the other variables were confounders.

3.1.2. Relationship between Engagement in Pacing and Physical Activity

Results of the relationship between engagement in pacing and physical activity, controlling for demographics and confounders (Table 4), revealed no association between engagement in pacing and physical activity ($\beta = -0.242$; $t = -1.61$, $p = 0.12$). None of the demographics and confounders was related to physical activity ($p \geq 0.05$).

Table 4. Hierarchical linear regression model showing the relationship between engagement in pacing and physical activity.

Variable	β	B	SE	df	t	p-Value
Age	−0.054	−5.555	15.028	3, 55	−0.370	0.713
Gender	0.084	198.685	327.197	3, 55	0.607	0.546
Body mass index	0.029	4.558	22.309	3, 55	0.204	0.839
Health-related quality of life	−0.069	−9.8272	0.678	2, 53	−0.475	0.637
Perceived risk of overactivity	0.067	86.563	181.272	2, 53	0.478	0.635
Engagement in pacing	−0.242	−3733.690	232.825	1, 52	−1.605	0.115

β, Standardized regression coefficients from the complete regression model accounting for all variables; B, unstandardized regression coefficients from the complete regression model accounting for all variables; df, degree of freedom; SE, standard error of B. Note: In this model, physical activity was the dependent variable, engagement in pacing was an independent variable, and the other variables were confounders.

For all analyses, the VIFs were low showing that there was no problem of multicollinearity (range: 1.04–1.30).

4. Discussion

This study explored relations of reported engagement in pacing with fatigue and physical activity, while controlling for demographics, health-related quality of life, and perceived risk of overactivity in adults with MS and found no associations between engagement in pacing and fatigue or and physical activity. These findings were similar to the findings of Murphy et al. [18] but did not support our hypothesis that engagement in pacing would be associated with low fatigue and high physical activity. Regarding the confounders, health-related quality of life was negatively related to fatigue. Descriptive statistics showed people with MS demonstrated clinically significant fatigue complaints, which was similar to studies evaluating fatigue in the MS population [32], high engagement in pacing and a high perceived risk of preventing overactivity. The total minutes of physical activity level reported by participants in our study is consistent with previous research involving people with MS [6,33]. The FSS score (5.43 ± 1.11) and percentage of participants reporting clinically significant fatigue (91.3%) in our study were comparable with those reported in other studies involving people with MS [1,34,35]. In their studies, Weiland et al. [34] and Hadgkiss et al. [35] reported median FSS score of 4.9 (IQR 3.2–6.1) with 65.6% of the sample reporting clinically significant fatigue. Similarly, Merkelbach et al. [1] reported a mean FSS score of 4.4 ± 1.6, with 58.75% of the sample reporting clinically significant fatigue.

Bivariate correlation analysis conducted prior to the primary analyses revealed a moderate negative association between fatigue and health-related quality of life, indicating high fatigue was associated with low health-related quality of life. Furthermore, there was a weak negative association between engagement in pacing and health-related quality of life, suggesting that high engagement in pacing was associated with low health-related quality life. Together, these findings suggest that without interventions, there appears to be no clear strategy for using physical activity to ameliorate fatigue symptoms and improve quality of life amongst people with MS. This underscores the need to explore the potential of guiding and advising people with MS regarding optimal pacing behaviour and to develop therapeutic interventions.

A possible explanation for the lack of associations between reported engagement in pacing and fatigue or physical activity after controlling for demographic and confounding variables, coupled with the clinically significant fatigue found in this study, may be multiplicity in persons' attitudes towards physical activity in relation to fatigue symptoms. People with MS who experience more disruption through fatigue in daily life may be consciously limiting their activities to prevent fatigue worsening, or exhibiting all-or-nothing behaviour, which is a lifestyle characterized by periods of overactivity (when feeling good) and as a consequence of that, feeling overtly fatigued afterwards, followed by long extensive rest periods to recover from residual symptoms or prevent symptoms re-occurring. For those consciously limiting their activities to prevent fatigue worsening, more engagement in pacing will most likely result in less physical activity, while for those exhibiting a lifestyle characterized by periods of overactivity and prolonged inactivity, more active engagement in pacing will most likely result in more physical activity, and thus when both attitudes are present in the subject population no relations between activity pacing and physical activity may be found.

This further highlights the importance to explore the natural use of activity pacing in relation to what we know from literature to help guide treatment efforts for people with MS. Tailored advice and goal-directed interventions on how to approach activity effectively, such as guidance on optimal use of pacing, might be beneficial for people with MS. For example, people who avoid physical activity in anticipation to fatigue might score high on engagement in pacing but may need advice to engage more in physical activity, and could be provided with a graded consistent program of physical activity to increase their health, as well as be given information and strategies to help change their beliefs that "I should do less if I am tired" or "symptoms are always a sign that I am damaging myself." Similarly, people who have developed an all-or-nothing behaviour style might need advice to be more aware of anticipatory ways of engaging in pacing to develop a consistent pattern of paced activity and rest.

To our knowledge this is the first study to tap into the experiences of people with MS during their daily routines and explore the associations between engagement in pacing, fatigue, and physical activity. Adequate management of fatigue might be essential to improve health and wellbeing in people with MS, based on the findings of this study and previous literature that revealed most people with MS experience high levels of fatigue throughout the day [31]. Though the sample size in this study was substantial for this population ($N = 80$), it would be useful to replicate these analyses in a larger sample to obtain more precise estimates of the model parameters while controlling for confounders. Furthermore, the adapted SQUASH, and the Activity Pacing and Risk of Overactivity Questionnaire used in this study are recent and have undergone limited validity and sensitivity testing, which may have influenced the study findings. Currently, further studies on the validity of these measurements and usage for the current purposes are being conducted. Although self-report measures are more feasible in population studies, they are susceptible to biases as they involve recalling activities (over days, weeks, or months) that could lead to underreporting or overreporting. Using an objective device would allow to examine more macro levels of activity and is warranted in future study.

To optimize generalizability within the population of people living with MS, this study was conducted solely in people with MS. Generalizability to other populations might therefore be limited, as findings may vary per condition [14]. Unfortunately, there was a lack of information on participants' MS type and MS disability in this study, which limits the ability to draw firm conclusions. These variables could influence the study findings. Lastly, the weak bivariate correlations between reported engagement in pacing and fatigue, and between reported engagement in pacing and physical activity found may have accounted for the lack of associations after controlling for demographics, health-related quality of life, and perceived risk of overactivity. It is worth noting that although participants received rehabilitation treatment as part of the larger multicenter study, a structured activity pacing program was not included and we do not think this has influenced the findings of this study. Future studies should further explore how engagement in pacing and perceived risk of overactivity relate to performance of activities of daily living, to allow for firm conclusions and help advice people with MS on how to engage in an active lifestyle. Additionally, exploratory studies on how activity pacing behaviour might affect physical activity, fatigue, and health-related quality of life over a longer period of time are warranted. Such studies should explore higher versus lower fatigue group in terms of clinical fatigue cut-off point (FSS > 4) or a median split, to help better understand associations.

5. Conclusions

This study examined the relationships between reported engagement in pacing and fatigue and physical activity in people with MS, while controlling for demographics, perceived risk of overactivity, and health-related quality of life. No associations were found between reported engagement in pacing and fatigue, or between reported engagement in pacing and physical activity. We found that low health-related quality of life was associated with high fatigue. People with MS might benefit from targeted interventions to better manage their fatigue and improve their health and wellbeing. Ascertaining engagement in pacing may be important to help tailor advice on optimal pacing behaviour for people with MS. There is a need to explore the potential of guiding and advising people with MS on activity pacing and develop therapeutic interventions.

Author Contributions: Conceptualization, U.S.A. and F.J.H.; Methodology, U.S.A., F.H., and B.L.S.; Validation, F.J.H., F.H., L.H.V.v.d.W., and R.D.; Formal Analysis, U.S.A., F.H., and B.L.S.; Resources, F.J.H., L.H.V.v.d.W., and R.D.; Data Curation, F.H. and B.L.S.; Writing—Original Draft Preparation, U.S.A. and F.J.H.; Writing—Review and Editing, U.S.A., F.J.H., F.H., B.L.S., L.H.V.v.d.W., and R.D.; Supervision, F.J.H., L.H.V.v.d.W., and R.D. All authors have read and agreed to the published version of the manuscript.

Funding: This research received no external funding.

Acknowledgments: The authors would like to thank all participants for their contribution to the ReSpAct study. Furthermore, we would like to thank the following organizations for their support in the ReSpAct study: Adelante zorggroep, Bethesda Ziekenhuis, De Trappenberg, De Vogellanden, Maasstad Ziekenhuis, Medisch Centrum Alkmaar, Militair Revalidatiecentrum Aardenburg, Revalidatiecentrum Leijpark, Revalidatiecentrum Reade, Revalidatie Friesland, Revant, Rijnlands Revalidatiecentrum, RMC Groot Klimmendaal, Scheper Ziekenhuis, Sint Maartenskliniek, Sophia Revalidatie, Tolbrug Revalidatie, ViaReva, and Stichting Onbeperkt Sportief.

Conflicts of Interest: The authors declare no conflict of interest.

Appendix A

Table A1. Factor loadings of the seven items of the Activity Pacing and Risk of Overactivity Questionnaire using Principal Component Analysis with oblique rotation.

Items	Factor 1	Factor 2
A. During the day I plan several moments to recover.	0.73 *	0.04
B. I perform my activities at a slow pace.	0.65 *	−0.13
C. When performing my activities, I take my fatigue into account.	0.79 *	0.00
D. When I'm engaged in an activity, I find it difficult to stop timely.	0.05	0.88 *
E. I alternate intensive activities with less intensive activities.	0.70 *	0.08
F. I divide my activities over the day.	0.74 *	−0.05
H. I find it hard to limit my activities.	−0.06	0.87

Factor 1: Engagement in pacing; Factor 2: Perceived risk of overactivity. * Loadings that can be explicitly assigned to a single factor (factor loading >0.40).

References

1. Merkelbach, S.; Schulz, H.; Kölmel, H.W.; Gora, G.; Klingelhöfer, J.; Dachsel, R.; Hoffmann, F.; Polzer, U. Fatigue, sleepiness, and physical activity in patients with multiple sclerosis. *J. Neurol.* **2011**, *258*, 74–79. [CrossRef]
2. Branas, P.; Jordan, R.; Fry-Smith, A.; Burls, A.; Hyde, C. Treatments for fatigue in multiple sclerosis: A rapid and systematic review. *Health Technol. Assess.* **2000**, *4*, 1–61. [CrossRef] [PubMed]
3. Bakshi, R. Fatigue associated with multiple sclerosis: Diagnosis, impact and management. *Mult. Scler.* **2003**, *9*, 219–227. [CrossRef] [PubMed]
4. Amato, M.P.; Ponziani, G.; Rossi, F.; Liedl, C.L.; Stefanile, C.; Rossi, L. Quality of life in multiple sclerosis: The impact of depression, fatigue and disability. *Mult. Scler.* **2001**, *7*, 340–344. [CrossRef] [PubMed]
5. Johansson, S.; Ytterberg, C.; Claesson, I.M.; Lindberg, J.; Hillert, J.; Andersson, M.; Holmqvist, L.W.; von Koch, L. High concurrent presence of disability in multiple sclerosis. *J. Neurol.* **2007**, *254*, 767–773. [CrossRef] [PubMed]
6. Motl, R.W.; McAuley, E.; Snook, E.M.; Scott, J.A. Validity of physical activity measures in ambulatory individuals with multiple sclerosis. *Disabil. Rehabil.* **2006**, *28*, 1151–1156. [CrossRef]
7. Motl, R.W.; McAuley, E.; Snook, E.M. Physical activity and multiple sclerosis: A meta-analysis. *Mult. Scler.* **2005**, *11*, 459–463. [CrossRef]

8. Andrews, N.E.; Strong, J.; Meredith, P.J. Activity pacing, avoidance, endurance, and associations with patient functioning in chronic pain: A systematic review and meta-analysis. *Arch. Phys. Med. Rehabil.* **2012**, *93*, 2109–2121. [CrossRef] [PubMed]
9. Roehrs, T.G.; Karst, G.M. Effects of an aquatics exercise program on quality of life measures for individuals with progressive multiple sclerosis. *J. Neurol. Phys. Ther.* **2004**, *28*, 63–71. [CrossRef]
10. Brurberg, K.G.; Odgaard-Jensen, J.; Price, J.R.; Larun, L. Exercise therapy for chronic fatigue syndrome. *Cochrane Database Syst. Rev.* **2017**, *4*, 144.
11. Nijs, J.; Van Eupen, I.; Vandecauter, J.; Augustinus, E.; Bleyen, G.; Moorkens, G.; Meeus, M. Can pacing self-management alter physical behaviour and symptom severity in chronic fatigue syndrome: A case series. *J. Rehabil. Res. Dev.* **2009**, *46*, 985–1069. [CrossRef] [PubMed]
12. National Institute for Health and Clinical Excellence (NICE). Clinical Guideline Chronic Fatigue Syndrome/Myalgic Encephalomyelitis or Encephalopathy: Diagnosis and Management of CFS/ME in Adults and Children. 2007. Available online: http://www.nice.org.uk/nicemedia/pdf/CG53NICEGuideline.pdf (accessed on 10 October 2016).
13. Antcliff, D.; Campbell, M.; Woby, S.; Keeley, P. Assessing the psychometric properties of an activity pacing questionnaire for chronic pain and fatigue. *Phys. Ther.* **2015**, *95*, 1274–1286. [CrossRef] [PubMed]
14. Abonie, U.S.; Edwards, M.; Hettinga, F.J. Optimising activity pacing to promote a physically active lifestyle in persons with a disability or chronic disease: A narrative review. *J. Sports Sci.* **2020**, *38*, 590–596. [CrossRef] [PubMed]
15. Abonie, U.S.; Sandercock, G.R.H.; Heesterbeek, M.; Hettinga, F.J. Effects of activity pacing in patients with chronic conditions associated with fatigue complaints: A meta-analysis. *Disabil. Rehabil.* **2020**, *42*, 613–622. [CrossRef]
16. Murphy, S.L.; Kratz, A.L. Activity pacing in daily life: A within-day analysis. *Pain* **2014**, *155*, 2630–2637. [CrossRef]
17. Murphy, S.L.; Smith, D.M.; Alexander, N.B. Measuring activity pacing in women with lower-extremity osteoarthritis: A pilot study. *Am. J. Occup. Ther.* **2008**, *62*, 329–334. [CrossRef]
18. Murphy, S.L.; Kratz, A.L.; Williams, D.A.; Geisser, M.E. The association between symptoms, pain coping strategies, and physical activity among people with symptomatic knee and hip osteoarthritis. *Front. Psychol.* **2012**, *3*, 326. [CrossRef]
19. Alingh, R.A.; Hoekstra, F.; van der Schans, C.P.; Hettinga, F.J.; Dekker, R.; van der Woude, L.H. Protocol of a longitudinal cohort study on physical activity behaviour in physically disabled patients participating in a rehabilitation counselling programme: ReSpAct. *BMJ Open* **2015**, *5*, e007591. [CrossRef]
20. Hoekstra, F.; Alingh, R.A.; van der Schans, C.P.; Hettinga, F.J.; Duijf, M.; Dekker, R.; van der Woude, L.H. Design of a process evaluation of the implementation of a physical activity and sport stimulation program in Dutch rehabilitation setting: ReSpAct. *Implement Sci.* **2014**, *9*, 127. [CrossRef]
21. Wendel-Vos, G.W.; Schuit, A.J.; Saris, W.H.; Kromhout, D. Reproducibility and relative validity of the short questionnaire to assess health-enhancing physical activity. *J. Clin. Epidemiol.* **2003**, *56*, 1163–1169. [CrossRef]
22. Krupp, L.B.; LaRocca, N.G.; Muir-Nash, J.; Steinberg, A.D. The fatigue severity scale. Application to patients with multiple sclerosis and systemic lupus erythematosus. *Arch. Neurol.* **1989**, *46*, 1121–1123. [CrossRef] [PubMed]
23. Selim, A.J.; Rogers, W.; Fleishman, J.A.; Qian, S.X.; Fincke, B.G.; Rothendler, J.A.; Kazis, L.E. Updated US population standard for the Veterans RAND 12-item Health Survey (VR-12). *Qual. Life Res.* **2009**, *18*, 43–52. [CrossRef] [PubMed]
24. Whitehead, L. The measurement of fatigue in chronic illness: A systematic review of unidimensional and multidimensional fatigue measures. *J. Pain Symptom Manag.* **2009**, *37*, 107–128. [CrossRef] [PubMed]
25. Smedal, T.; Beiske, A.G.; Glad, S.B.; Myhr, K.M.; Aarseth, J.H.; Svensson, E.; Gjelsvik, B.; Strand, L.I. Fatigue in multiple sclerosis: Associations with health-related quality of life and physical performance. *Eur. J. Neurol.* **2011**, *18*, 114–120. [CrossRef] [PubMed]
26. Arends, S.; Hofman, M.; Kamsma, Y.P.; van der Veer, E.; Houtman, P.M.; Kallenberg, C.G.; Spoorenberg, A.; Brouwer, E. Daily physical activity in ankylosing spondylitis: Validity and reliability of the IPAQ and SQUASH and the relation with clinical assessments. *Arthritis Res. Ther.* **2013**, *15*, R99. [CrossRef]

27. Wagenmakers, R.; van den Akker-Scheek, I.; Groothoff, J.W.; Zijlstra, W.; Bulstra, S.K.; Kootstra, J.W.; Wendel-Vos, G.W.; van Raaij, J.J.; Stevens, M. Reliability and validity of the short questionnaire to assess health-enhancing physical activity (SQUASH) in patients after total hip arthroplasty. *BMC Musculoskelet. Disord.* **2008**, *9*, 141. [CrossRef]
28. Hays, R.D. *RAND 36 Health Status Inventory*; Harcourt Brace & Company: New York, NY, USA, 1998.
29. Ware, J.E., Jr.; Kosinski, M.; Keller, S.D. A 12-time short form health survey: Construction of scales and preliminary tests of reliability and validity. *Med. Care* **1996**, *34*, 220–233. [CrossRef]
30. IBM Corp. *IBM SPSS Statistics for Windows*; Version 23; IBM Corp: Armonk, NY, USA, 2015.
31. Enoka, R.M.; Duchateau, J. Translating fatigue to human performance. *Med. Sci. Sports Exerc.* **2016**, *48*, 2228–2238. [CrossRef]
32. Heine, M.; van den Akker, L.E.; Blikman, L.; Hoekstra, T.; Van Munster, E.; Verschuren, O.; Visser-Meily, A.; Kwakkel, G.; de Groot, V.; Beckerman, H.; et al. Real-time assessment of fatigue in patients with multiple sclerosis: How does it relate to commonly used self-report fatigue questionnaires? *Arch. Phys. Med. Rehabil.* **2016**, *97*, 1887–1894. [CrossRef]
33. Gosney, J.L.; Scott, J.A.; Snook, E.M.; Motl, R.W. Physical activity and multiple sclerosis: Validity of self-report and objective measures. *Fam. Commun. Health* **2007**, *30*, 144–150. [CrossRef]
34. Weiland, T.J.; Jelinek, G.A.; Marck, C.H.; Hadgkiss, E.J.; van der Meer, D.M.; Pereira, N.G.; Taylor, K.L. Clinically Significant Fatigue: Prevalence and Associated Factors in an International Sample of Adults with Multiple Sclerosis Recruited via the Internet. *PLoS ONE* **2015**, *10*, e0115541. [CrossRef] [PubMed]
35. Hadgkiss, E.J.; Jelinek, G.A.; Weiland, T.J.; Pereira, N.G.; Marck, C.H.; van der Meer, D.M. Methodology of an International Study of People with Multiple Sclerosis Recruited through Web 2.0 Platforms: Demographics, Lifestyle, and Disease Characteristics. *Neurol. Res. Int.* **2013**, *2013*, 580596. [PubMed]

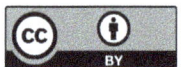

© 2020 by the authors. Licensee MDPI, Basel, Switzerland. This article is an open access article distributed under the terms and conditions of the Creative Commons Attribution (CC BY) license (http://creativecommons.org/licenses/by/4.0/).

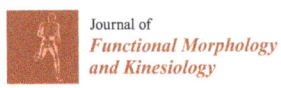

Article

Adjuvant Therapy Reduces Fat Mass Loss during Exercise Prescription in Breast Cancer Survivors

Gabriele Mascherini *, Benedetta Tosi, Chiara Giannelli, Elena Ermini, Leonardo Osti and Giorgio Galanti

Dipartimento di Medicina Sperimentale e Clinica, Università degli Studi di Firenze, 50134 Firenze, Italy; benedetta.tosi@unifi.it (B.T.); CHIARA_GIANNELLI@libero.it (C.G.); ermini.elena@gmail.com (E.E.); leo.osti@alice.it (L.O.); giorgio.galanti@unifi.it (G.G.)
* Correspondence: gabriele.mascherini@unifi.it; Tel.: +39-3396895925

Received: 26 May 2020; Accepted: 11 July 2020; Published: 15 July 2020

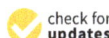

Abstract: Improvements in cancer care over the years have increased the numbers of cancer survivors. Therefore, quality of life, fat mass management and physical activity are growing areas of interest in these people. After the surgical removal of a breast cancer, adjuvant therapy remains anyway a common strategy. The aim of this study was to assess how adjuvant therapy can affect the effectiveness of an unsupervised exercise program. Forty-two women were enrolled (52.0 ± 10.1 years). Assessments performed at baseline and after six months of exercise prescription were body composition, health-related quality of life, aerobic capacity by Six-Minute Walk Test, limbs strength by hand grip and chair test and flexibility by sit and reach. Statistical analyses were conducted by ANOVA tests and multiple regression. Improvements in body composition, physical fitness and quality of life (physical functioning, general health, social functioning and mental health items) were found. The percentage change in fat mass has been associated with adjuvant cancer therapy (intercept = −0.016; b = 8.629; $p < 0.05$). An unsupervised exercise prescription program improves body composition, physical fitness and health-related quality of life in breast cancer survivors. Adjuvant therapy in cancer slows down the effectiveness of an exercise program in the loss of fat mass.

Keywords: physical activity; oncology; unsupervised exercise; lifestyle; exercise prescription

1. Introduction

Breast cancer is the most commonly diagnosed cancer in women around the world, the second cause of cancer death in female population of developed countries (198,000 deaths in 2012) and the first cause of cancer death in Italian women (12,274 deaths in 2015) [1].

The importance of lifestyle in the etiopathogenesis of this disease is well-demonstrated [2]. After a cancer diagnosis, patients report a feeling of fatigue that can result from the side effects of the treatment or from the cancer itself. This promotes an increase in physical inactivity, which increases the likelihood of incurring overweight and obesity [3]. The excess weight condition is associated with a low-grade systemic inflammation that promotes the development of insulin resistance, atherosclerosis and tumor growth, even in cancer survivors. This may explain the association between cancer and cardiovascular / metabolic diseases [4]. The impact of comorbidities on all-causes mortality in breast cancer survivors is remarkable [5].

Women with a diagnosis of breast cancer may experience disease and treatment-related adverse physiological and psychosocial effects at short and long-term [6]. After surgery, adjuvant therapy in the form of hormone therapy, chemotherapy or target molecular therapy is generally considered [1].

These therapeutic choices seem to promote short-term body composition changes by increasing body water and long-term in terms of increasing fat mass [7].

In order to reduce chronic inflammation, fat mass reduction is one of the most important outcome of any exercise prescription program, as it can contribute to decrease recurrence risk and to increase disease-free and overall survival [8]. Exercise training in breast cancer survivors can maintain or improve VO$_2$peak, significantly improved lean body mass, upper and lower body strength [9].

Cancer can also negatively affect in terms of health-related quality of life (HRQoL) and psychosocial and physical function [6]. It is well known that physical activity has small-to-moderate beneficial effects on HRQoL, as well as on emotional or perceived physical and social function, anxiety, cardiorespiratory fitness [6,9] of breast cancers survivors during and after adjuvant treatment. HRQoL, whose improvements are considered a prognostic indicator of overall survival in cancer patients, normally worsens after cancer diagnosis and during cancer treatments [10,11].

Physical activity interventions may help to improve prognosis and may alleviate the adverse effects of adjuvant therapy in terms of body composition and HRQoL. Home-based exercise program demonstrated both a short and long-term effectiveness in physical function and body composition parameters [12,13].

This study aimed to:

- Evaluate how adjuvant therapy can influence the effectiveness of an unsupervised exercise program in terms of fat loss, analyzing how different therapeutic choices can have a different effect;
- Verify the effectiveness of an unsupervised exercise program on health-related quality of life in breast cancer survivors.

2. Materials and Methods

2.1. Subjects

The data of this observational study were collected from September 2015 to September 2017. The Breast Unit of the Careggi University Hospital selected and enrolled patients. After, they began the exercise prescription program at the Sports Medicine Center of the same University Hospital.

2.1.1. Inclusion Criteria

The patients included in this study met the following inclusion criteria: (1) female, (2) from 21 to 65 years old, (3) physiological or pharmacological induced menopausal (4) history of surgery for breast cancer, (5) no participation in other training programs or no regular attendance at health clubs.

2.1.2. Exclusion Criteria

The participants were excluded from the study if they said they were physically unable to participate in the treatment protocol or if changes in their physical activity behavior were contraindicated. The participants were also excluded if they were taking antipsychotic medication or undergoing any weight-loss strategy.

The participants were required to provide their written consent prior to their inclusion in the study as well as a letter of approval to participate from their oncologist and sports physician. All procedures performed in studies involving human participants were in accordance with the ethical standards of the institutional and national research committee and with the 1964 Helsinki declaration.

2.2. Procedures

The program at Sport Medicine Center consisted in:

- First visit (T0): history, cardiac evaluation, lifestyle assessment, body composition analysis, physical fitness parameters related to health and health-related quality of life.

- Follow-up visits (every 30 days): body composition analysis and health-related physical fitness parameters.
- six months follow-up visit (T5) body composition analysis, physical fitness parameters related to health and health-related quality of life.

2.2.1. Medical History and Cardiac Evaluation

All patients were evaluated before starting the program to exclude any contraindication and thus provide eligibility to physical exercise. They underwent assessment by health questionnaire (to exclude any family history for chronic or metabolic diseases, anticancer therapies, comorbidity and any symptoms), physical examination, ECG at rest and 2-dimensional echocardiography to exclude chemotherapy-induced cardiotoxicity.

2.2.2. Lifestyle Assessment

Lifestyle was assessed at the beginning of the program to evaluate the spontaneous physical activity [14]. An accelerometer (armband model MF-SW, display model DD100, SenseWear®, BodyMedia®, Pittsburgh, Pennsylvania, USA) on the non-dominant arm of the patients to be kept for one week. The parameters provided by the specific software were:

- Total energy expenditure in Kcal per day;
- Kcal > 3 METS expenses per day;
- PAL (physical activity level) defined as total energy expenditure/resting metabolic rate;
- Steps per day;
- Time spent in sedentary behaviors 1 to 1.49 METs (min);
- Light physical activity 1.5 to 2.99 metabolic equivalent of task (METs) mild physical activity (min);
- Moderate physical activity 3 to 5.99 METs (min);
- Vigorous physical activity > 6 METs (min);

2.2.3. Body-Composition Analysis

The same researcher evaluated body composition, measuring anthropometric parameters, skinfold for subcutaneous adipose tissue and bio impedance for fat-free mass [15].

Measures of weight were approximated to the nearest 0.1 kg, those of height to the nearest 0.5 cm (Seca GmbH &Co., Hamburg, Germany), BMI was then calculated (kg/m^2). Waist, hip, operated and not operated arm (in case of bilateral surgery, non-dominant arm values were considered as "operated") circumferences were also measured using a measuring tape (Holtain Limited, Crosswell, UK, 1.5 m flexible tape). Waist–hip ratio was calculated [16].

Triceps, biceps, subscapular and supra-iliac skinfolds were measured by calipers (Holtain, Limited Tanner/Whitehouse skinfold caliper, Crosswell, UK) and sum (mm) of the four skinfold sites was calculated [17].

Bio impedance analysis (BIA 101 Sport edition, Akern, Florence, Italy) provided the values of resistance (Rz) and reactance (Xc) [18]: from these two the phase angle (PA), the amounts of total body water (TBW), extracellular water (ECW), intracellular water (ICW), fat free mass (FFM), body cell mass (BCM), muscle mass (MM) and fat mass (FM) were obtained.

2.2.4. Health-Related Physical Fitness Parameters

The six minute walk test (6MWT) assessed cardiovascular fitness, because most daily life activities are performed at submaximal levels of exertion, this test may better reflect the functional exercise level for daily physical activities [19]. The parameters recorded during 6MWT were distance covered (6 MWD), peak heart rate with a heart rate monitor, systolic and diastolic blood pressure at rest and at the end of the test and self-perception of effort (CR10) [20].

Muscle fitness evaluation were performed with easily executable and reproducible tests in an outpatient setting such as sit & reach for flexibility [21], the hand grip test to estimate the overall static strength of the upper limbs with both arms [22] and the chair test to assess the strength of the lower limbs [23].

2.2.5. Health-Related Quality of Life Assessment

Health-related quality of life was assessed by administering the SF-36 questionnaire. This is a validated tool that measures eight health concepts [24]: physical functioning (PF), role limitations due to physical health problems (RP), bodily pain (BP), general health (GH), vitality (VT), social functioning (SF), role limitations due to personal or emotional problems (RE) and mental health (MH) perceptions. Scores for each domain range from 0 to 100, with a higher score defining a more favorable health state [25].

2.2.6. Exercise Prescription

Exercise program were prescribed at the end of the first visit following American College of Sports Medicine guidelines [26]. The program did not include supervised exercise. The combination of duration and weekly session aerobic training (such as walking, cycling or jogging) were established starting from thirty minutes five times per week (150 min per week) while intensity were establish in terms of heart rate and perceived of effort based on 6MWT. In addition, a target of number daily step were provided. At the end of each aerobic exercise sessions, flexibility exercise have been recommended. resistance training has been suggested twice per week with 8 exercises involving the main muscle groups, performed for 3 sets with 10 repetitions. The exercises were chosen based on the possibility of being performed safely at home (such as bodyweight squat and glute bridge for the lower limbs, lateral raise and biceps curl for the upper limbs). At the end of each visit, the prescribed exercise program was described. Furthermore, for resistance exercise, a demonstration was performed by qualified personnel in physical exercise followed by repetition by the patient as a learning test. Exercise program were individually updated every follow-up visit following the results of the assessments.

2.3. Statistical Analysis

The data were expressed as mean ± standard deviation. The Shapiro–Wilk test was used to assess the normal distribution of variables. one-way ANOVA was performed to evaluate the variations of the body composition and fitness parameters between baseline and final study values (T0-T5). The Cohen's d effect size (ES) was calculated to determine the magnitude of effect. ES was assessed using the following criteria: small < 0.20, medium < 0.50 and large < 0.80.

The answers to the SF-36 questions were recorded and recalibrated to obtain a raw score that was then converted into the correspondent percentage score. A paired Student's t-test was used to establish differences between baseline and six months SF-36 parameters.

A multiple linear regression was used to assess the relationship between the percentage change in fat mass during the program calculate as $[(\Delta \text{ T5-T0 FM/FM T0}) \cdot 100)]$ and three potential predictors as: (1) adjuvant cancer therapy, (2) fat mass at baseline and (3) age at baseline.

One-way ANOVA and the Bonferroni's test for multiple comparison were used to establish the potential differences among the different kinds of adjuvant therapy in term of change of fat mass. Therapy was considered with four subgroups: hormone therapy only, chemotherapy and/or target therapy, any combination of therapies, no therapy. The data were analyzed using SPSS-IBM 20 (SPSS, Inc., Chicago, IL, USA). The statistical significance threshold was set at a p-value = 0.05.

3. Results

A group of 42 women (age 52.0 ± 10.1 years) were considered eligible for the study and were then enrolled. All the patients had been diagnosed with a stage IIIC or inferior breast cancer and started the program after the surgery: 48% had undergone unilateral mastectomy with lymphadenectomy, 19% unilateral quadrantectomy with lymphadenectomy, 19% unilateral quadrantectomy, 12% bilateral mastectomy with bilateral lymphadenectomy, 2% bilateral mastectomy with unilateral lymphadenectomy.

Specific neoplastic therapy was: 15 took hormone therapy (tamoxifen and aromatase inhibitors), 9 underwent chemotherapy and/or target therapy (anthracycline and trastuzumab), 9 combined hormone therapy with chemotherapy and/or target therapy, and 9 did not undergo any adjuvant cancer therapy.

3.1. Lifestyle Assessment

The results of lifestyle assessment were:

- Total energy expenditure 2210.0 ± 336.0 kcal/day;
- Kcal> 3 METS 338.2 ± 263.6 kcal/day;
- Steps per day 8224.5 ± 2846.3;
- PAL 1.55 ± 0.18;
- Sedentary behaviors 16.5 ± 3.10 h/day;
- Light physical activity 4.9 ± 1.7 h/day;
- Moderate physical activity 78 ± 12.0 min/day;
- Vigorous physical activity 2.4 ± 0.02 min/day.

3.2. Body Composition Analysis

Baseline anthropometric parameters assessment defined an overweight sample (BMI T0 = 27.3 ± 4.20 kg/m^2) and 30% was obese (BMI ≥ 30.0 kg/m^2; Table 1).

Table 1. Anthropometrics and skinfold parameters during 6 months follow-up.

	T0	T5	Δ T5-T0	F Value	ANOVA	ES
Weight (kg)	71.9 ± 10.8	68.7 ± 10.1	−3.2 ± 2.3	6.47	<0.001	1.36
BMI (kg/m^2)	27.3 ± 4.2	26.1 ± 3.9	−1.2 ± 0.9	6.12	<0.001	1.34
Waist circ. (cm)	90.2 ± 10.8	85.3 ± 9.8	−4.9 ± 4.0	6.02	<0.001	1.22
Hip circ. (cm)	106.1 ± 9.1	102.1 ± 7.1	−4.0 ± 3.9	5.76	<0.001	1.02
Waist/hip	0.85 ± 0.069	0.83 ± 0.06	−0.01 ± 0.04	0.23	NS	0.36
Operated arm circ. (cm)	31.8 ± 3.4	29.5 ± 2.6	−2.4 ± 1.7	5.43	<0.001	1.39
Not operated arm circ. (cm)	31.5 ± 3.4	29.4 ± 2.7	−2.1 ± 2.1	4.32	<0.001	0.99
Biceps skinfold (mm)	16.9 ± 8.1	13.8 ± 6.5	−3.1 ± 5.0	4.01	<0.001	0.61
Triceps skinfold (mm)	27.1 ± 5.7	23.5 ± 5.6	−3.6 ± 2.9	5.21	<0.001	1.26
Subscapular skinfold (mm)	25.5 ± 7.9	22.2 ± 7.1	−3.3 ± 3.9	4.55	<0.001	0.82
Supra–iliac skinfold (mm)	24.3 ± 8.9	21.0 ± 7.7	−3.3 ± 7.1	3.42	0.032	0.46
Skinfold sum (mm)	93.8 ± 25.5	80.5 ± 22.6	−13.3 ± 12.5	6.12	<0.001	1.06

During the six months of follow-up the patients lost weight progressively, getting close to overweight threshold (BMI T5 = 26.1 ± 3.87 kg/m^2), others anthropometric parameters decreased, in particular waist circumference dropped below the cardio metabolic risk threshold. Skinfold thickness data and bio impedance analysis showed that weight loss is principally imputable to a fat mass loss and secondarily to extracellular water loss (Table 1).

On the contrary, body cellular mass and intracellular water did not show any significant change. The amount of total body water and fat free mass reduced is attributable to extracellular mass loss (Table 2).

Table 2. Bio-impedance parameters during 6 months follow-up.

	T0	T5	Δ T5-T0	F Value	ANOVA	ES
PA (°)	5.2 ± 0.7	5.3 ± 0.7	0.2 ± 0.7	0.31	NS	0.23
TBW (L)	35.0 ± 3.3	34.2 ± 3.3	−0.9 ± 1.8	3.12	0.025	0.48
ECW (L)	17.5 ± 1.9	16.8 ± 1.9	−0.7 ± 1.5	4.22	<0.001	0.50
ICW (L)	17.5 ± 2.3	17.4 ± 2.2	−0.1 ± 1.6	0.68	NS	0.08
FFM (kg)	46.7 ± 4.7	45.7 ± 4.4	−1.0 ± 2.9	4.88	0.002	0.36
BCM (kg)	23.1 ± 3.3	22.9 ± 3.1	−0.1 ± 2.1	1.08	NS	0.06
FM (kg)	25.0 ± 8.1	22.6 ± 7.2	−2.4 ± 3.4	4.23	<0.001	0.72

Legend: PA—phase angle; TBW—total body water; ECW—extra cellular water; ICW—intra cellular water; FFM—fat free mass; BCM—body cellular mass; FM—fat mass.

3.3. Health-Related Physical Fitness Parameters

All the physical fitness parameters improved progressively. Moreover, the values at rest of systolic (SBP), diastolic (DBP) blood pressures and mean arterial pressure (MAP) decreased significantly (Table 3).

Table 3. Physical fitness parameters related to health during 6 months follow-up.

	T0	T5	Δ T5-T0	F Value	ANOVA	ES
Chair test (reps)	14.5 ± 3.8	18.3 ± 4.3	3.8 ± 2.6	8.12	<0.001	1.45
Hand Gr. op. arm (kg)	24.3 ± 4.8	26.5 ± 4.5	2.2 ± 4.5	3.55	0.012	0.48
Hand Gr. not op. arm (kg)	24.2 ± 4.6	26.4 ± 4.3	2.2 ± 3.1	4.78	<0.001	0.72
Sit and reach test (cm)	2.6 ± 9.3	8.5 ± 7.1	5.8 ± 6.0	6.02	<0.001	0.97
6 MWD (m)	518.6 ± 133.0	584.8 ± 97.2	66.2 ± 107.2	4.28	<0.001	0.62
HR rest (bpm)	75.6 ± 13.5	73.5 ± 10.5	−2.1 ± 11.8	3.92	0.015	0.18
SBP rest (mmHg)	117 ± 15.1	110 ± 12.7	−6.4 ± 13.4	3.04	0.048	0.48
DBP rest (mmHg)	76.1 ± 11.3	70.6 ± 8.7	−5.5 ± 9.70	4.11	0.013	0.57
MAP rest (mmHg)	89.7 ± 11.5	83.9 ± 9.2	−5.8 ± 9.8	4.11	0.012	0.59

Legend: HR—heart rate; SBP—systolic blood pressure; DBP—diastolic blood pressure; MAP—mean arterial pressure.

3.4. Health-Related Quality of Life Assessment

As far as the health-related quality of life is concerned, all the eight health concepts measured by the SF-36 questionnaire were improved: those found in PF, GH, SF and MH scales registered a significant improvement, and those found in BP, VT and RE scales were, anyhow, very close to significance threshold (Table 4).

Table 4. Results of health-related quality of life parameters measured by social functioning (SF)-36 questionnaire.

	T0	T5	Δ T5-T0	p-Value
PF (%)	72.7 ± 24.6	83.7 ± 17.1	11.0 ± 15.9	<0.001
RP (%)	61.3 ± 39.1	65.5 ± 37.4	4.17 ± 33.5	0.43
BP (%)	61.0 ± 25.8	67.4 ± 22.0	6.40 ± 30.3	0.18
GH (%)	64.7 ± 20.4	69.1 ± 18.9	4.43 ± 6.97	<0.001
VT (%)	52.7 ± 18.4	57.4 ± 16.7	4.64 ± 15.0	0.051
SF (%)	60.5 ± 24.5	67.6 ± 22.9	7.08 ± 20.1	0.027
RE (%)	56.4 ± 43.2	65.9 ± 33.3	9.53 ± 37.7	0.11
MH (%)	63.4 ± 14.8	67.3 ± 12.5	3.90 ± 10.7	0.022

Legend: PF—physical functioning; RP—role limitations due to physical health problems; BP—bodily pain; GH—general health; VT—vitality; SF—social functioning; RE—role limitations due to personal or emotional problems; MH—mental health perceptions.

3.5. Relationship between Adjuvant Cancer Therapy and Changes in Fat Mass

The association between percentage change in fat mass and the three potential predictors were ($R^2 = 0.52$; MSE = 5.73): adjuvant cancer therapy coefficients = 8.63, $p < 0.05$; fat mass at baseline coefficients = −0.32, $p = 0.36$; age at baseline coefficients = 0.18, p = 0.26. In particular, this association between change in fat mass and adjuvant cancer therapy one-way ANOVA shows these differences existed between no therapy subgroup and any other subgroup (F = 5.12, $p = 0.018$, ES = 0.68), but no differences existed among these last subgroups of therapy:

- No therapy shows a fat mass reduction −16.5% ± 13.2%;
- Hormone therapy shows a fat mass reduction −6.5% ± 9.1%;
- Chemotherapy and/or target therapy shows a fat mass reduction −6.8% ± 10.4%;
- Hormone therapy + chemotherapy and/or target therapy shows a fat mass reduction −6.9% ± 9.0%.

Therefore, adjuvant cancer therapy was negatively associated with fat mass loss observed between baseline and six months.

4. Discussion

This study confirmed the effectiveness in terms of body composition and physical fitness of unsupervised exercise program in breast cancer survivor [12,13].

After the surgical removal of a breast cancer, adjuvant therapy is a common strategy. However, higher breast cancer risk with hormone replacement therapy is particularly evident among lean women, in postmenopausal women who are not taking exogenous hormones; general obesity is a significant predictor for breast cancer recurrence. Moreover, increased plasma cholesterol leads to accelerated tumor formation and exacerbates their aggressiveness [6].

The sample of the present study shows the anthropometric and lifestyle parameters in line with other studies already present [27]; these characteristics do not appear to guarantee a healthy level of cardiorespiratory fitness. Therefore, these patients should carry out a regular exercise program in order to ensure an improvement in health-related physical fitness parameters [28].

The therapeutic efficacy of the physical exercise is now consistent and demonstrated by systematic reviews and meta-analyses in the context of secondary and tertiary prevention of breast cancer [29,30]. Physical activity in breast cancer survivors may be more effective at modifying serum IGF-1 levels in women who are not taking tamoxifen [31], on the insulin pathway may be more pronounced for obese or sedentary women [32]. A marginal effect of physical activity in terms of decreasing circulating levels of biomarkers of inflammation in particular (CRP) [33] and in circulating levels of markers of cell-mediated immunity [34]. In this context, unsupervised training strategy could be an option in a physical exercise therapy perspective.

One of the aims of the study was to evaluate the influence of adjuvant therapy on the effectiveness of an exercise program on fat loss and how different therapeutic choices can have a different effect. A recent review [35] reports that exercise is effective in reducing fat mass during adjuvant therapy in breast cancer. However, the difference in efficacy between the different therapeutic strategies and the comparison of efficacy with those who do not perform any adjuvant therapy is not specified. The results of multiple regression in this study confirm the effectiveness of the exercise in reducing fat mass during adjuvant therapy without however any difference between the various therapeutic choices. However, those who did not have an adjuvant treatment regimen reported a greater reduction in fat mass than those who had an adjuvant therapy in place.

Health-related quality of life results are consistent with those shown in other studies where SF-36 questionnaire was used [36]. SF-36 is indeed a questionnaire that can be applied to many different clinical situations and that measures health concepts (particularly RE and MH) that can be influenced by a large number of factors (including changes in cancer therapies, that can signify changes in side effects associated with them). Anyway, the documented correlation between the other six scales and physical health perception, together with the improvements observed in body composition and physical fitness, justify the attribution to the program of at least a part of the improvements that is proportional to the correlation coefficient of each scale. Indeed, the lack of significance for RP, BP, VT and RE scales is almost surely due to the difference in statistical power that characterizes the eight scales: with a larger sample, significance would be obtained. Regarding RE and MH scales instead, it is only possible to consider that women have on average improved: this cannot be random, supporting the thesis that the program is capable of improving these two health concepts as well. It is important to notice that a major score in BP, RP and RE scales corresponds, respectively to minor pain, less limitation due to physical health problems and less limitation due to personal or emotional problems.

Poor prognosis in cancer survivors is associated with reduced levels of fitness, increased fat mass and decreased lean body mass [37]. Aerobic and resistance exercises prescription is capable of improving body composition, physical fitness and health-related quality of life of breast cancer survivors. American College of Sport Medicine's guidelines [26] provide rough indications about intensity, duration and frequency of aerobic, resistance and flexibility exercises, highlighting the importance of considering a large number of factors (age, exercise endurance, drugs taken, cancer stage) to prescribe exercise safely and effectively. Anyhow, the ultimate goal of any exercise prescription program for cancer survivors is to induce long-term modifications in patients' lifestyle, in order to reduce recurrence risk, cancer mortality and all causes of mortality [38]. From this perspective, unsupervised exercise programs can ensure good adherence in cancer survivors [39], even in those undergoing adjuvant treatments.

The present study shows strengths. First, all the subjects belonged to the same Breast Unit, therefore they undergone to surgery from the same surgeon group. Second, the sample receive the exercise program from the same Sport Medicine Center by the same specialist, therefore the methodology was standardized.

The study has limitations. The first limit is in the observational nature of an outpatient exercise prescription program; therefore, the intervention of the researcher was limited, and some adjustments were not possible. Second, body composition changes did not take into account the energy intake; therefore, the results have a reduced generalizability.

Larger samples are needed to confirm these results and future research directions could be the association between adjuvant therapies and the loss of fat mass assessed also with lipid blood values in addition to subcutaneous fat.

5. Conclusions

The results shown in this study demonstrate that an unsupervised exercised prescription program produces mid-term improvements in body composition, physical fitness and health-related quality of life of breast cancer survivors. Adjuvant therapy in cancer slows down the effectiveness of an exercise program in the loss of fat mass. Longer-term follow-up studies are needed to establish the real capacity of this training strategy to induce long-term lifestyle changes.

Author Contributions: Conceptualization, G.M. and G.G.; methodology, L.O.; validation, G.G., L.O. and G.M.; formal analysis, L.O. and G.M.; investigation, E.E.; data curation, G.M. and L.O.; writing—original draft G.M., C.G. and B.T.; project administration, C.G. and B.T. All authors have read and agreed to the published version of the manuscript.

Funding: This research received no external funding

Conflicts of Interest: The authors declare no conflicts of interest.

References

1. I Numeri del Cancro in Italia. Available online: https://www.aiom.it/wp-content/uploads/2018/10/2018_NumeriCancro-operatori.pdf (accessed on 15 May 2020).
2. Engin, A. Obesity-associated Breast Cancer: Analysis of risk factors. *Adv. Exp. Med. Biol.* **2017**, *960*, 571–606. [CrossRef] [PubMed]

3. Pedersen, B.K. The diseasome of physical inactivity–and the role of myokines in muscle–fat cross talk. *J. Physiol.* **2009**, *587*, 5559–5568. [CrossRef] [PubMed]
4. Kerr, J.; Anderson, C.; Lippman, S.M. Physical activity, sedentary behaviour, diet, and cancer: An update and emerging new evidence. *Lancet Oncol.* **2017**, *18*, e457–e471. [CrossRef]
5. Ahern, T.P.; Lash, T.L.; Thwin, S.S.; Silliman, R.A. Impact of acquired comorbidities on all-cause mortality rates among older breast cancer survivors. *Med. Care.* **2009**, *47*, 73–79. [CrossRef] [PubMed]
6. Pedersen, B.; Delmar, C.; Lörincz, T.; Falkmer, U.; Grønkjær, M. Investigating Changes in Weight and Body Composition Among Women in Adjuvant Treatment for Breast Cancer: A Scoping Review. *Cancer Nurs.* **2019**, *42*, 91–105. [CrossRef] [PubMed]
7. Lahart, I.M.; Metsios, G.S.; Nevill, A.M.; Carmichael, A.R. Physical activity for women with breast cancer after adjuvant therapy. *Cochrane Database Syst. Rev.* **2018**, *2018*, CD011292. [CrossRef] [PubMed]
8. Azrad, M.; Demark-Wahnefried, W. The association between adiposity and breast cancer recurrence and survival: A review of the recent literature. *Curr. Nutr. Rep.* **2014**, *3*, 9–15. [CrossRef] [PubMed]
9. Kirkham, A.A.; Bland, K.A.; Sayyari, S.; Campbell, K.L.; Davis, M.K. Clinically Relevant Physical Benefits of Exercise Interventions in Breast Cancer Survivors. *Curr. Oncol. Rep.* **2016**, *18*, 12. [CrossRef] [PubMed]
10. Quinten, C.; Coens, C.; Mauer, M.; Comte, S.; Sprangers, M.A.; Cleeland, C.; Osoba, D.; Bjordal, K.; Bottomley, A. Baseline quality of life as a prognostic indicator of survival: A meta-analysis of individual patient data from EORTC clinical trials. *Lancet Oncol.* **2009**, *10*, 865–871. [CrossRef]
11. Montazeri, A. Quality of life data as prognostic indicators of survival in cancer patients: An overview of the literature from 1982 to 2008. *Health Qual. Life Outcomes.* **2009**, *7*, 102. [CrossRef] [PubMed]
12. Mascherini, G.; Tosi, B.; Giannelli, C.; Grifoni, E.; Degl'innocenti, S.; Galanti, G. Breast cancer: Effectiveness of a one-year unsupervised exercise program. *J. Sports Med. Phys. Fit.* **2019**, *59*, 283–289. [CrossRef] [PubMed]
13. Mascherini, G.; Giannelli, C.; Ghelarducci, G.; Degl'Innocenti, S.; Petri, C.; Galanti, G. Active lifestyle promotion with home-based exercise in breast cancer survivors. *J. Hum. Sport Exerc.* **2017**, *12*, 119–128. [CrossRef]
14. Stefani, L.; Mascherini, G.; Scacciati, I.; De Luca, A.; Maffulli, N.; Galanti, G. Positive effect of the use of accelerometry on lifestyle awareness of overweight hypertensive patients. *Asian J. Sports Med.* **2013**, *4*, 241–248. [CrossRef] [PubMed]
15. Mascherini, G.; Petri, C.; Galanti, G. Integrated total body composition and localized fat-free mass assessment. *Sport Sci. Health.* **2015**, *11*, 217. [CrossRef]
16. Welborn, T.A.; Dhaliwal, S.S.; Bennett, S.A. Waist–hip ratio is the dominant risk factor predicting cardiovascular death in Australia. *Med. J. Aust.* **2003**, *179*, 580–585. [CrossRef] [PubMed]
17. Esparza-Ros, F.; Vaquero-Cristóbal, R.; Marfell-Jones, M. *International Protocol for Anthropometric Assessment*; International Society for the Advancement of Kinanthropometry (ISAK): Murcia, Spain, 2019.
18. Foster, K.F.; Lukaski, H.C. Whole-body impedance—what does it measure? *Am. J. Clin. Nutr.* **1996**, *64*, 388S–396S. [CrossRef] [PubMed]
19. Solway, S.; Brooks, D.; Lacasse, Y.; Thomas, S. A qualitative systematic overview of the measurement properties of functional walk tests used in the cardiorespiratory domain. *Chest* **2001**, *119*, 256–270. [CrossRef] [PubMed]
20. Arney, B.E.; Glover, R.; Fusco, A.; Cortis, C.; de Koning, J.J.; van Erp, T.; Jaime, S.; Mikat, R.P.; Porcari, J.P.; Foster, C. Comparison of RPE (Rating of Perceived Exertion) Scales for Session RPE. *Int. J. Sports Physiol. Perform.* **2019**, *14*, 994–996. [CrossRef] [PubMed]
21. Mayorga-Vega, D.; Merino-Marban, R.; Viciana, J. Criterion related validity of sit and reach tests for estimating hamstring and lumbar extensibility: A meta analysis. *J. Sports Sci. Med.* **2014**, *13*, 1–14. [PubMed]
22. Gomes, P.R.L.; Junior, I.F.F.; Da Silva, C.B.; Gomes, I.C.; Rocha, A.P.R.; Salgado, A.S.I.; Carmo, E.M.D. Short term changes in handgrip strength, body composition, and lymphedema induced by breast cancer surgery. *Rev. Bras. Ginecol. Obstet.* **2014**, *36*, 244–250. [CrossRef] [PubMed]
23. Calabró, M.A.; Lee, J.M.; Saint-Maurice, P.F.; Yoo, H.; Welk, G.J. Validity of physical activity monitors for assessing lower intensity activity in adults. *Int. J. Behav. Nutr. Phys. Act.* **2014**, *11*, 119. [CrossRef] [PubMed]
24. Hart, V.; Trentham-Dietz, A.; Berkman, A.; Fujii, M.; Veal, C.; Hampton, J.; Gangnon, R.; Newcomb, P.A.; Gilchrist, S.C.; Sprague, B.L. The association between post-diagnosis health behaviors and long-term quality of life in survivors of ductal carcinoma in situ: A population-based longitudinal cohort study. *Qual. Life Res.* **2018**, *27*, 1237–1247. [CrossRef] [PubMed]

25. Apolone, G.; Mosconi, P. The Italian SF-36 Health Survey: Translation, validation and norming. *J. Clin. Epidemiol.* **1998**, *51*, 1025–1036. [CrossRef]
26. Pescatello, L.S.; Riebe, D.; Arena, R.; American College of Sports Medicine. *ACSM's Guidelines for Exercise Testing and Prescription*, 9th ed.; Lippincott Williams & Wilkins: Baltimore, MD, USA, 2014.
27. Santos-Lozano, A.; Ramos, J.; Alvarez-Bustos, A.; Cantos, B.; Alejo, L.B.; Pagola, I.; Soria, A.; Maximiano, C.; Fiuza-Luces, C.; Soares-Miranda, L.; et al. Cardiorespiratory fitness and adiposity in breast cancer survivors: Is meeting current physical activity recommendations really enough. *Support. Care Cancer* **2018**, *26*, 2293–2301. [CrossRef] [PubMed]
28. Gómez, A.M.; Martínez, C.; Fiuza-Luces, C.; Herrero, F.; Pérez, M.; Madero, L.; Ruiz, J.R.; Lucia, A.; Ramírez, M. Exercise training and cytokines in breast cancer survivors. *Int. J. Sports Med.* **2011**, *32*, 461–467. [CrossRef] [PubMed]
29. Battaglini, C.L.; Mills, R.C.; Phillips, B.; Lee, J.T.; E Story, C.; Nascimento, M.G.; Hackney, A.C. Twenty-five years of research on the effects of exercise training in breast cancer survivors: A systematic review of the literature. *World J. Clin. Oncol.* **2014**, *10*, 177–190. [CrossRef] [PubMed]
30. Speck, R.M.; Courneya, K.S.; Mâsse, L.C.; Duval, S.; Schmitz, K.H. An update of controlled physical activity trials in cancer survivors: A systematic review and meta-analysis. *J. Cancer Surviv.* **2010**, *4*, 87–100.
31. Fairey, A.S.; Courneya, K.S.; Field, C.J.; Bell, G.J.; Jones, L.W.; Mackey, J.R. Randomized controlled trial of exercise and blood immune function in postmenopausal breast cancer survivors. *J. Appl. Physiol.* **2005**, *98*, 1534–1540. [CrossRef] [PubMed]
32. A Ligibel, J.; Campbell, N.; Partridge, A.; Chen, W.Y.; Salinardi, T.; Chen, H.; Adloff, K.; Keshaviah, A.; Winer, E.P. Impact of a mixed strength and endurance exercise intervention on insulin levels in breast cancer survivors. *J. Clin. Oncol.* **2008**, *26*, 907–912. [CrossRef] [PubMed]
33. Fairey, A.S.; Courneya, K.S.; Field, C.J.; Bell, G.J.; Jones, L.W.; Martin, B.S.; Mackey, J.R. Effect of exercise training on C-reactive protein in postmenopausal breast cancer survivors: A randomized controlled trial. *Brain Behav. Immun.* **2005**, *19*, 381–388. [CrossRef] [PubMed]
34. Irwin, M.L.; Varma, K.; Alvarez-Reeves, M.; Cadmus, L.; Wiley, A.; Chung, G.G.; DiPietro, L.; Mayne, S.T.; Yu, H. Randomized controlled trial of aerobic exercise on insulin and insulin-like growth factors in breast cancer survivors: The Yale Exercise and Survivorship study. *Cancer Epidemiol. Biomarkers Prev.* **2009**, *18*, 306–313. [CrossRef] [PubMed]
35. Lee, J.; Lee, M.G. Effects of Exercise Interventions on Breast Cancer Patients During Adjuvant Therapy: A Systematic Review and Meta-analysis of Randomized Controlled Trials. *Cancer Nurs.* **2020**, *43*, 115–125. [CrossRef] [PubMed]
36. Navigante, A.; Morgado, P.C. Does physical exercise improve quality of life of advanced cancer patients? *Curr. Opin. Support Palliat Care.* **2016**, *10*, 306–309. [CrossRef] [PubMed]
37. Clark, W.; Siegel, E.M.; Chen, Y.A.; Zhao, X.; Parsons, C.M.; Hernandez, J.M.; Weber, J.; Thareja, S.; Choi, J.; Shibata, D. Quantitative measures of visceral adiposity and body mass index in predicting rectal cancer outcomes after neoadjuvant chemoradiation. *J. Am. Coll. Surg.* **2013**, *216*, 1070–1081. [CrossRef] [PubMed]
38. Pedersen, B.K.; Saltin, B. Exercise as medicine-evidence for prescribing exercise as therapy in 26 different chronic diseases. *Scand J. Med. Sci. Sports.* **2015**, *25*, 1–72. [CrossRef] [PubMed]
39. Stefani, L.; Klika, R.; Mascherini, G.; Mazzoni, F.; Lunghi, A.; Petri, C.; Petreni, P.; Di Costanzo, F.; Maffulli, N.; Galanti, G. Effects of a home-based exercise rehabilitation program for cancer survivors. *J. Sports Med. Phys. Fitness.* **2019**, *59*, 846–852. [CrossRef] [PubMed]

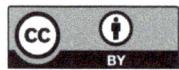

© 2020 by the authors. Licensee MDPI, Basel, Switzerland. This article is an open access article distributed under the terms and conditions of the Creative Commons Attribution (CC BY) license (http://creativecommons.org/licenses/by/4.0/).

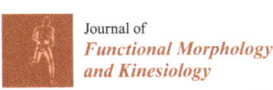

Review

Adapted Physical Activity to Ensure the Physical and Psychological Well-Being of COVID-19 Patients

Grazia Maugeri [1] and Giuseppe Musumeci [1,2,3,*]

1. Department of Biomedical and Biotechnological Sciences, Human, Histology and Movement Science Section, University of Catania, via S. Sofia 87, 95123 Catania, Italy; graziamaugeri@unict.it
2. Research Center on Motor Activities (CRAM), University of Catania, via S. Sofia 87, 95123 Catania, Italy
3. Department of Biology, Sbarro Institute for Cancer Research and Molecular Medicine, College of Science and Technology, Temple University, Philadelphia, PA 19122, USA
* Correspondence: g.musumeci@unict.it; Tel.: +39-095-378-2043

Abstract: The novel coronavirus disease 2019 (COVID-19) has been responsible for a global pandemic involving massive increases in the daily numbers of cases and deaths. Due to the emergency caused by the pandemic, huge efforts have been made to develop COVID-19 vaccines, the first of which were released in December 2020. Effective vaccines for COVID-19 are needed to protect the population, especially healthcare professionals and fragile individuals, such as older people or chronic-disease-affected patients. Physical exercise training generally has health benefits and assists in the prevention of several chronic diseases. Moreover, physical activity improves mental health by reducing anxiety, depression, and negative mood and improving self-esteem. Therefore, the present review aims to provide a detailed view of the literature, presenting updated evidence on the beneficial effects of adapted physical activity, based on personalized and tailor-made exercise, in preventing, treating, and counteracting the consequences of COVID-19.

Keywords: COVID-19; prevention; physical activity; inactivity; home-based exercise; mental health; psychological well-being

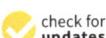

Citation: Maugeri, G.; Musumeci, G. Adapted Physical Activity to Ensure the Physical and Psychological Well-Being of COVID-19 Patients. *J. Funct. Morphol. Kinesiol.* **2021**, *6*, 13. https://doi.org/10.3390/jfmk6010013

Received: 25 November 2020
Accepted: 27 January 2021
Published: 29 January 2021

Publisher's Note: MDPI stays neutral with regard to jurisdictional claims in published maps and institutional affiliations.

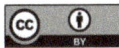

Copyright: © 2021 by the authors. Licensee MDPI, Basel, Switzerland. This article is an open access article distributed under the terms and conditions of the Creative Commons Attribution (CC BY) license (https://creativecommons.org/licenses/by/4.0/).

1. Introduction

The social effects caused by the global spread and pandemic of SARS-CoV-2 is having unimaginable consequences that the world has never faced in past decades. After the WHO declared SARS-CoV-2 a health emergency, the world responded quickly to "flatten the curve" or limit the spread of the virus by banning travel and closing non-essential businesses and educational institutions, as well stopping all kinds of large gatherings. In this first phase of the pandemic, around half of the world's population was under full or partial lockdown to limit the spread of the deadly virus [1]. The unprecedented restrictions prompted by the raging SARS CoV-2 pandemic halted a wide variety of economic activities throughout the world. Day by day, the need for essential healthcare equipment increased in parallel with the increase of infected patients and death tolls. More than 100 countries closed their borders and worldwide air travel demand plummeted just after the announcement of the pandemic by the WHO. This severely impacted the world's supply chain and international trade [2]. Economists agreed that there would be an enormous negative impact on global economic development due to COVID-19, which would possibly plunge the world economy into a deep recession [3]. Therefore, after this initial lockdown period, a second phase started, involving the partial reopening of the economy. However, increasing cases and limited numbers of intensive care beds have caused public health authorities in Europe to re-impose temporary lockdowns.

Global health authorities have been informed by epidemic and infectious disease specialists, who have faced the present health emergency by taking cues from past epidemics. However, we now know that the story of COVID-19 cannot be compared to past epidemics. Besides the high direct mortality for such a contagious acute disease, COVID-19 has placed extreme pressure on healthcare systems, altering access to health services of patients living with other pathologies, such as non-communicable diseases (NCDs). Moreover, such NCDs (e.g., diabetes mellitus, hypertension, cerebrovascular disease, coronary artery disease, chronic obstructive pulmonary disease) have been shown to predict poor prognosis in patients with COVID-19. SARS-CoV-2 and NCDs are clustering within social groups according to patterns of socioeconomic inequality that are deeply embedded in our societies. Limiting the harm caused by SARS-CoV-2 will demand that far greater attention is paid to NCDs and socioeconomic inequality than has previously been done. The aggregation of these diseases against a background of social and economic disparity aggravates the adverse effects of each separate disease. COVID-19 is not a pandemic or simple comorbidity—it is a syndemic [4]. Addressing COVID-19 means addressing hypertension, obesity, malnutrition, diabetes, cardiovascular and chronic respiratory diseases, cancer, and psychological and neurodegenerative disorders. Paying more attention to NCDs and socioeconomic inequality should be a strategic plan for both rich and poor nations in order to limit the harm caused by SARS-CoV-2.

The worldwide spread of SARS-CoV-2 infection has caused governments of various countries to take swift and unprecedented protective measures, including placing cities in lockdown and closing places where large gatherings would occur. Quarantine has radically changed the daily habits of the entire population, requiring people to practice "social distancing". For example, in Italy, the Italian Ministry of Education (MIUR) decided to invest huge resources in special desks to promote higher interpersonal distance in classrooms to avoid the risk of infection [5]. Although such strategies have contained the COVID-19 outbreak, the prolonged self-isolation has deeply affected active lifestyles, leading healthy individuals and athletes to states of physical inactivity, with related consequences of hypomobility and inactivity-associated disorders, such as a reduction in maximal oxygen consumption (VO2max), endurance capacity, loss of muscle strength and mass, overweight, and decrease joint lubrification [6–9]. Just a few days of a sedentary lifestyle are sufficient to induce fiber denervation, insulin resistance, and low-grade systemic inflammation [10].

The positive effects of regular physical activity on general health are well known in the field of modern medicine. Physical activity counteracts cardiovascular vulnerability, inflammation, muscle atrophy, bone and cartilage loss or degeneration, and the reduction of aerobic capacity [11,12]. Physical exercise is also closely related to cognitive function and neurodegenerative disorders by inducing cellular and molecular processes underlying neurogenesis and synaptogenesis cascade, which enhance learning, memory, and brain plasticity [13,14]. These effects are extremely important, especially in light of new evidence showing brain damage among the consequences of COVID-19, including delirium, stroke, and brain inflammation. Moreover, adapted physical activity ameliorates one's self-esteem and provides a sense of well-being by reducing the development of mental disorders [15]. In light of this evidence, the purpose of this narrative mini-review is to summarize the beneficial effects of the adapted physical activity performed before-, during-, and post-infection of COVID-19. To this end, four databases were used: PubMed, Scopus, Web of Science, and Google Scholar. The last search was conducted on 30 December 2020. The following keywords and combinations thereof were used: "exercise", "physical activity", "adapted physical activity", "physical exercise", "SARS-CoV-2", "SARS CoV-2 pandemic", "COVID-19 pandemic". The initial study selection was performed via title and abstract screening. Duplicates were removed. The full texts of the selected articles were carefully read and analyzed in order to extract the appropriate data from each text.

2. The Beneficial Effects of Physical Activity before COVID-19 Infection

The development of COVID-19 is strictly linked to the interaction between SARS-CoV-2 and the host's immune system. The virus affects the response of the immune system, leading to leukopenia with high levels of pro-inflammatory mediators. Several studies have shown that in mild cases of COVID-19, macrophages of pulmonary tissue are able to counteract SARS-CoV-2 and the innate and adaptive immune responses are able to fight viral replication. In contrast, severe cases of COVID-19 provoke a storm of pro-inflammatory cytokines and a lymphopenia state [16]. This "hyper inflammation" is characterized by aberrant pathogenic T cells and inflammatory monocytes, which are rapidly activated and produce a large number of cytokines, thus inducing the inflammatory storm [16]. Moreover, some COVID-19-affected patients have developed acute demyelinating encephalomyelitis (ADEM), without showing respiratory symptoms [17,18], and in some cases Guillan-Barrè syndrome has been diagnosed, characterized by nerve damage [19]. The SARS-CoV-2 virus is usually not present in patients' cerebrospinal brain fluid. Therefore, it is possible to speculate that brain inflammation is caused by the immune system and that the neurological complications of COVID-19 might be provoked by the deregulated immune response rather than the virus itself [20]. The role of physical exercise in improving immune response has largely been demonstrated. Moderate and adapted physical activity increases the anti-inflammatory cytokines, immunoglobulins, and immune cells in circulation, as well as the anti-pathogenic activity of macrophages [21]. In this way, physical exercise may cause reductions of the burden of pathogen and the abnormal inflammatory cells that damage the lungs [22]. Interestingly, COVID-19-affected patients have reported higher levels of cytokines, such as TNF-α, IFN-γ, IL-1β, and IL-6, as compared to healthy subjects [23,24]. Moreover, the expression levels of these pro-inflammatory cytokines to be appeared directly related to the severity of the patient's condition, confirming that the activation of the inflammatory process is linked to disease severity [23,24].

The implementation of the physical activity program could play a key role in counteracting the imbalance in antiviral immunity, protecting the individual against inflammation induced by COVID-19. According to WHO recommendations, all adults should undertake 150–300 min of moderate-intensity, 75–150 min of vigorous-intensity physical activity, or some equivalent combination of moderate-intensity and vigorous-intensity aerobic physical activity per week. Among children and adolescents, an average of 60 min/day of moderate–vigorous-intensity aerobic physical activity across the week provides health benefits. These guidelines recommend regular muscle-strengthening activity for all age groups [25]. The adapted physical activity comprises an exercise program designed in a personalized way in order to adapt to the physiological characteristics and the state of health of each subject. Its beneficial role in low-grade chronic inflammation was demonstrated in both the periphery and in the brain [26]. During its practices, stress hormones and microglia proliferation are decreased. Moreover, physical activity attenuates the release of proinflammatory cytokines through the modulation of anti-inflammatory cytokines, such as IL-1Ra, IL-6, and IL-10, as well as cytokine inhibitors, such as cortisol, prostaglandin E2, and soluble receptors against TNF and IL-2 [26]. Considering that adapted physical activity has shown several benefits for most chronic diseases and microbial infections with preventive and therapeutic effects, in the pre-infection phase, it may represent an important tool to prevent COVID-19 infection [27]. Furthermore, several pieces of evidence supported the direct relationship between exercise and psychological well-being. Individuals who practice regular physical activity ameliorate one's self-esteem and provide a sense of well-being, leading to reduced depressive and anxiety symptoms [28,29]. This plethora of positive effects is due to the involvement of the hypothalamic–pituitary–adrenal (HPA) axis and the endogenous opioid system, both of which are implied in anxiety, stress, depression, and emotional responses [30,31]. In addition, regular exercise promotes the release of several trophic factors, including brain-derived neurotrophic factor (BDNF), which exerts a positive role in both anxiety and depressive disorders [32]. Quarantine and physical isolation measures may have had long-lasting and wide-ranging negative psychosocial impacts, which may have been amplified by a reduction in physical activity levels. Several works have demonstrated the negative impacts of decreased physical activity on psychological well-being [33–36]. In particular, a decrease in the amount of physical activity is associated with higher levels of perceived stress and anxiety [33]. A study performed on older adults showed that those who met the global recommendations on physical activeness had higher levels of resilience and lower levels of depressive symptoms [36]. The promotion of resilience during the COVID-19 pandemic is a crucial aspect for patients, considering that it is linked to positive emotions in stressful situations, locus of control, self-efficacy, optimism, and better quality of life (physical and psychological) [35]. In particular, Lesser and Nienhuis [33] reported that individuals who were more physically active showed greater mental health scores, whereas inactive subjects before the COVID-19 pandemic who became more active during the lockdown exhibited lower levels of anxiety. Moreover, a cross-national study between Germany, Italy, Russia, and Spain, showed that individuals with depression symptoms are at risk of developing a worse psychological condition during the current Covid-19 pandemic; instead, physical activity counteract such negative effects [37]. Interestingly, the profoundly negative impacts on psychological health and well-being in the population seem to be higher in females and young adults [32].

3. Adapted Physical Activity Program during COVID-19 Infection

Considering the clinical characteristics of COVID-19, infected patients, who are compelled to rest in bed, are not able to perform normal activities of daily life or perform regular physical activity. Nevertheless, considering the multiple positive effects caused by exercise, adapted physical activity in all phases of recovery of patients (Figure 1) represents an important strategy to attenuate the decline in cognition function and to improve physical and psychological well-being in individuals affected by COVID-19. When treating patients—and given the intensive medical management involved for some COVID-19 patients, including prolonged protective lung ventilation, immobility, sedation, and treatment with neuromuscular blocking agents—in the acute phase it is possible to adopt only passive types of exercise performed by physiotherapists or kinesiologists, such as whole-body vibration (WBV) exercise and passive range-of-motion (pROM) exercises. In the post-acute phase, however, physiotherapists or kinesiologists can organize bed-based exercise programs (e.g., flexion and extension of the limbs and trunk) and assist patients to mobilize independently to stand-up and perform normal daily functions according to the Barthel index, such as washing, eating, and so on. Other adapted physical activities, comprising passive, active-assisted, active, or resisted joint range-of-motion exercises, are fundamental to restore and improve respiratory and cardiocirculatory functions, joint integrity, range-of-motion, muscle strength, and mental condition. During the day, hospitalized patients should perform the exercises alone by following a guided self-assessment for people with an acquired disability, which should be administered by physiotherapists or kinesiologists. This progressive approach as well as the known effects of general well-being can help keep patients busy and attenuate feelings of depression due to complete immobility. Regaining self-mobility can result in the patient acquiring better self-esteem and a strong response to depression.

Pneumonia, a severe complication of the virus, has been shown to induce cognitive decline due to sustained hypoxia [38,39]. Moreover, pneumonia patients were found to possess high levels of pro-inflammatory cytokines, leading to neuroinflammation and neurodegeneration [40]. Therefore, the positive influence of physical activity on cognitive performance is fundamental to accelerate the subsequent full recovery of COVID-19 patients. In fact, different studies have demonstrated that physical exercise enhances the neuronal activity and hippocampal neurogenesis essential for cognition [41,42]. Furthermore, adapted physical activity for COVID-19 patients represents a key psychological support. Exercise stimulates the cholinergic, dopaminergic, and serotonergic systems, enhancing mood by reducing depression, anxiety, and panic attacks [6,34]. In light of these positive effects on mental and psychological health, adapted or tailor-made exercises in COVID-19-affected individuals should be considered.

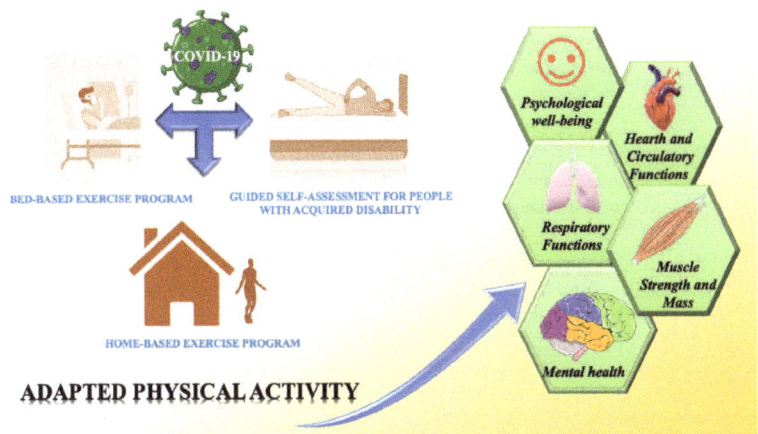

Figure 1. Health benefits from regular adapted physical activity in COVID-19-affected patients.

4. Adapted Physical Activity Program Post COVID-19 Infection

Once completely well, to maintain mental and physical well-being, it is vital for infected individuals to gradually resume physical activity and exercise with an adapted or tailor-made home-based exercise program administered by a sport scientist. The goal is to return to pre-infection levels of fitness. In this phase, the effects of physical activity on the brain trigger systemic influences on the entire body. Moreover, exercise promotes the release of endorphins, which enhance psychological well-being, favoring faster recovery and a return to normal life. Beyond conventional exercises to improve physical conditions, different activities are recommended to enhance psychological well-being, such as listening to music, reading or listening to a book, watching TV, playing cards, table games, and the utilization of "exergames" (i.e., active video games). These activities allow patients to keep busy, reducing depression. In particular, the use of exergames can positively affect motivation and self-efficacy by inducing physical activity practice [43]. Exergames use action and motion sensors, which allow the patient to be physically active, simulating several sport types, such as cycling, running, walking, rowing, and swimming. Moreover, the patient can also play exergames with a partner, favoring interaction and communication between them [44]. Another potentially beneficial activity during the patient recovery could be yoga. The practice of this discipline promotes endogenous melatonin secretion, positively affecting sleep quality, anxiety, and depressive disorders [45].

To allow the complete recovery of individuals, an interesting approach with several therapeutic benefits is Nordic walking. This activity is typically carried out in "healthy" environments, such as mountain, sea, and countryside settings, and is suitable for people of all ages. Nordic walking is useful for adapted motor re-education, especially for COVID-19 patients who have developed respiratory, metabolic, cardiovascular, and walking problems. Through the use of a specific pair of poles, Nordic walking engages the upper body muscles, and relative to normal walking would increase the overall energy expenditure [46]. Furthermore, since poles are held in both hands, the knees and joints are subjected to less stress; therefore, Nordic walking might be recommended in degenerative cartilage disorders, such as osteoarthritis [47], as it improves motor function and strength [48]. Interestingly, Nordic walking e-poles developed by Gabel, the Italian leading manufacturer in this area, are able to acquire the primary parameters that characterize the proper movement technique, providing feedback regarding the patient's performance and assisted walking. Nordic walking strengthens cognitive function, attention, and executive functions by positively affecting patient quality-of-life [49]. It is noteworthy that Nordic walking also exerts a positive effect on an individual's psychological well-being. Compared to normal walking, a previous study showed that this discipline elicited significant psychological improvements, ameliorating depression and sleep disturbance [50].

5. Conclusions

The SARS-CoV-2 virus represents the major societal challenge, with important repercussions for people's mental and physical health. The beneficial effects of physical exercise in improving quality of life and well-being have been extensively documented. An adapted physical activity program may represent an important factor to prevent COVID-19 infection, as well as a useful complementary tool to improve the physical and psychological outcomes of COVID-19-affected patients. A suitable exercise program may strengthen the respiratory system, providing immune protection in the long term and reducing treatment costs. Furthermore, in the post-infection phase, an adapted or tailor-made home-based exercise program ensures a faster return to pre-infection fitness by enhancing self-esteem and resilience to stress and reducing anxiety and depression.

Funding: This work was supported by the University Research Project Grant (PIACERI Found—NATURE-OA—2020–2022), Department of Biomedical and Biotechnological Sciences (BIOMETEC), University of Catania, Italy.

Acknowledgments: Our thoughts go out to all the victims of this pandemic and their families.

Conflicts of Interest: The authors declare no conflict of interest.

References

1. Koh, D. COVID-19 lockdowns throughout the world. *Occup. Med.* **2020**, *70*, kqaa073. [CrossRef]
2. Mishra, M.K. The World after COVID-19 and Its Impact on Global Economy. 2020. Available online: https://www.econstor.eu/handle/10419/215931 (accessed on 26 January 2021).
3. Fernandes, N. *Economic Effects of Coronavirus Outbreak (Covid-19) on the World Economy*; SSRN: Rochester, NY, USA, 2020.
4. Horton, R. Offline: COVID-19 is not a pandemic. *Lancet* **2020**, *396*, 874. [CrossRef]
5. Bergamin, M.; Musumeci, G. The utility of Anti-Covid-19 desks in Italy, doubts and criticism. *J. Funct. Morphol. Kinesiol.* **2021**, *6*, 2. [CrossRef] [PubMed]
6. Ravalli, S.; Musumeci, G. Coronavirus outbreak in Italy. Physiological benefits of home-based exercise during pandemic. *J. Funct. Morphol. Kinesiol.* **2020**, *5*, 31. [CrossRef] [PubMed]
7. Giustino, V.; Parroco, A.M.; Gennaro, A.; Musumeci, G.; Palma, A.; Battaglia, G. Physical activity levels and related energy expenditure during covid-19 quarantine among the sicilian active population: A cross-sectional online survey study. *Sustainability* **2020**, *12*, 4356. [CrossRef]
8. Paoli, A.; Musumeci, G. Elite athletes and covid-19 lockdown: Future health concerns for an entire sector. *J. Funct. Morphol. Kinesiol.* **2020**, *5*, 30. [CrossRef]
9. Methnani, J.; Amor, D.; Yousfi, N.; Bouslama, A.; Omezzine, A.; Bouhlel, E. Sedentary behavior, exercise and COVID-19: Immune and metabolic implications in obesity and its comorbidities. *J. Sports Med. Phys. Fit.* **2020**. [CrossRef]
10. Narici, M.; De Vito, G.; Franchi, M.; Paoli, A.; Moro, T.; Marcolin, G.; Grassi, B.; Baldassarre, G.; Zuccarelli, L.; Biolo, G.; et al. Impact of sedentarism due to the COVID-19 home confinement on neuromuscular, cardiovascular and metabolic health: Physiological and pathophysiological implications and recommendations for physical and nutritional countermeasures. *Eur. J. Sport Sci.* **2020**, *12*, 1–22. [CrossRef]
11. Castrogiovanni, P.; Di Rosa, M.; Ravalli, S.; Castorina, A.; Guglielmino, C.; Imbesi, R.; Vecchio, M.; Drago, F.; Szychlinska, M.A.; Musumeci, G. Moderate physical activity as a prevention method for knee osteoarthritis and the role of synoviocytes as biological key. *Int. J. Mol. Sci.* **2019**, *20*, 511. [CrossRef]
12. Szychlinska, M.A.; Castrogiovanni, P.; Trovato, F.M.; Nsir, H.; Zarrouk, M.; Lo Furno, D.; Di Rosa, M.; Imbesi, R.; Musumeci, G. Physical activity and Mediterranean diet based on olive tree phenolic compounds from two different geographical areas have protective effects on early osteoarthritis, muscle atrophy and hepatic steatosis. *Eur. J. Nutr.* **2019**, *58*, 565–581. [CrossRef]
13. Maugeri, G.; D'agata, V. Effects of physical activity in amyotrophic lateral sclerosis. *J. Funct. Morphol. Kinesiol.* **2020**, *5*, 29. [CrossRef] [PubMed]
14. Van Praag, H.; Christie, B.R.; Sejnowski, T.J.; Gage, F.H. Running enhances neurogenesis, learning, and long-term potentiation in mice. *Proc. Natl. Acad. Sci. USA* **1999**, *96*, 13427–13431. [CrossRef] [PubMed]
15. Van Minnen, A.; Hendriks, L.; Olff, M. When do trauma experts choose exposure therapy for PTSD patients? A controlled study of therapist and patient factors. *Behav. Res. Ther.* **2010**, *48*, 312–320. [CrossRef] [PubMed]
16. Cao, X. COVID-19: Immunopathology and its implications for therapy. *Nat. Rev. Immunol.* **2020**, *20*, 269–270. [CrossRef] [PubMed]
17. Parsons, T.; Banks, S.; Bae, C.; Gelber, J.; Alahmadi, H.; Tichauer, M. COVID-19-associated acute disseminated encephalomyelitis (ADEM). *J. Neurol.* **2020**, *267*, 2799–2802. [CrossRef] [PubMed]

18. Paterson, R.W.; Brown, R.L.; Benjamin, L.; Nortley, R.; Wiethoff, S.; Bharucha, T.; Jayaseelan, D.L.; Kumar, G.; Raftopoulos, R.E.; Zambreanu, L.; et al. The emerging spectrum of COVID-19 neurology: Clinical, radiological and laboratory findings. *Brain* **2020**, *143*, 3104–3120. [CrossRef]
19. Padroni, M.; Mastrangelo, V.; Asioli, G.M.; Pavolucci, L.; Abu-Rumeileh, S.; Piscaglia, M.G.; Querzani, P.; Callegarini, C.; Foschi, M. Guillain-Barré syndrome following COVID-19: New infection, old complication? *J. Neurol.* **2020**, *267*, 1877–1879. [CrossRef]
20. Wu, Y.; Xu, X.; Chen, Z.; Duan, J.; Hashimoto, K.; Yang, L.; Liu, C.; Yang, C. Nervous system involvement after infection with COVID-19 and other coronaviruses. *Brain Behav. Immun.* **2020**, *87*, 18–22. [CrossRef]
21. Di Rosa, M.; Castrogiovanni, P.; Musumeci, G. The synovium theory: Can exercise prevent knee osteoarthritis? the role of "mechanokines", a possible biological key. *J. Funct. Morphol. Kinesiol.* **2019**, *4*, 11. [CrossRef]
22. Nieman, D.C.; Wentz, L.M. The compelling link between physical activity and the body's defense system. *J. Sport Health Sci.* **2019**, *8*, 201–217. [CrossRef]
23. Liu, J.; Li, S.; Liu, J.; Liang, B.; Wang, X.; Wang, H.; Li, W.; Tong, Q.; Yi, J.; Zhao, L.; et al. Longitudinal characteristics of lymphocyte responses and cytokine profiles in the peripheral blood of SARS-CoV-2 infected patients. *EBioMedicine* **2020**, *55*, 102763. [PubMed]
24. Merad, M.; Martin, J.C. Pathological inflammation in patients with COVID-19: A key role for monocytes and macrophages. *Nat. Rev. Immunol.* **2020**, *20*, 355–362. [CrossRef] [PubMed]
25. Bull, F.C.; Al-Ansari, S.S.; Biddle, S.; Borodulin, K.; Buman, M.P.; Cardon, G.; Carty, C.; Chaput, J.P.; Chastin, S.; Chou, R.; et al. World Health Organization 2020 guidelines on physical activity and sedentary behaviour. *Br. J. Sports Med.* **2020**, *54*, 1451–1462. [CrossRef] [PubMed]
26. Petersen, A.M.W.; Pedersen, B.K. The anti-inflammatory effect of exercise. *J. Appl. Physiol.* **2005**, *98*, 1154–1162. [CrossRef]
27. Fernández-Lázaro, D.; González-Bernal, J.J.; Sánchez-Serrano, N.; Navascués, L.J.; Ascaso-Del-Río, A.; Mielgo-Ayuso, J. Physical Exercise as a Multimodal Tool for COVID-19: Could It Be Used as a Preventive Strategy? *Int. J. Environ. Res. Public Health* **2020**, *17*, 8496. [CrossRef]
28. Scully, D.; Kremer, J.; Meade, M.M.; Graham, R.; Dudgeon, K. Physical exercise and psychological well-being: A critical review. *Br. J. Sports Med.* **1998**, *32*, 111–120. [CrossRef]
29. Fox, K.R. The influence of physical activity on mental well-being. *Publ. Health Nutr.* **1999**, *2*, 411–418. [CrossRef]
30. Crews, D.J.; Landers, D.M. A meta-analytic review of aerobic fitness and reactivity to psychosocial stressors. *Med. Sci. Sports Exerc.* **1987**, *19* (Suppl. 5), S114–S120. [CrossRef]
31. Bodnar, R.J.; Klein, G.E. Endogenous opiates and behavior: 2003. *Peptides* **2004**, *25*, 2205–2256. [CrossRef]
32. Phillips, C. Brain-derived neurotrophic factor, depression, and physical activity: Making the neuroplastic connection. *Neural. Plast.* **2017**, *7260130*. [CrossRef]
33. Lesser, I.A.; Nienhuis, C.P. The impact of COVID-19 on physical activity behavior and well-being of Canadians. *Int. J. Environ. Res. Public Health* **2020**, *17*, 3899. [CrossRef]
34. Maugeri, G.; Castrogiovanni, P.; Battaglia, G.; Pippi, R.; D'Agata, V.; Palma, A.; Di Rosa, M.; Musumeci, G. The impact of physical activity on psychological health during Covid-19 pandemic in Italy. *Heliyon* **2020**, *6*, e04315. [CrossRef] [PubMed]
35. Duncan, G.E.; Avery, A.R.; Seto, E.; Tsang, S. Perceived change in physical activity levels and mental health during COVID-19: Findings among adult twin pairs. *PLoS ONE* **2020**, *15*, e0237695. [CrossRef] [PubMed]
36. Carriedo, A.; Cecchini, J.A.; Fernandez-Rio, J.; Méndez-Giménez, A. COVID-19, Psychological well-being and physical activity levels in older adults during the nationwide lockdown in spain. *Am. J. Geriatr. Psychiatry* **2020**, *28*, 1146–1155. [CrossRef] [PubMed]
37. Brailovskaia, J.; Cosci, F.; Mansueto, G.; Miragall, M.; Herrero, R.; Baños, R.M.; Krasavtseva, Y.; Kochetkov, Y.; Margraf, J. The association between depression symptoms, psychological burden caused by Covid-19 and physical activity: An investigation in Germany, Italy, Russia, and Spain. *Psychiatry Res.* **2020**, *295*, 113596. [CrossRef]
38. McCoy, J.G.; McKenna, J.T.; Connolly, N.P.; Poeta, D.L.; Ling, L.; McCarley, R.W.; Strecker, R.E. One week of exposure to intermittent hypoxia impairs attentional set-shifting in rats. *Behav. Brain Res.* **2010**, *210*, 123–126. [CrossRef]
39. Nunnari, G.; Sanfilippo, C.; Castrogiovanni, P.; Imbesi, R.; Volti, G.L.; Barbagallo, I.; Musumeci, G.; Di Rosa, M. Network perturbation analysis in human bronchial epithelial cells following SARS-CoV2 infection. *Exp. Cell Res.* **2020**, *395*, 112204. [CrossRef]
40. Danese, A.; Moffitt, T.E.; Pariante, C.M.; Ambler, A.; Poulton, R.; Caspi, A. Elevated inflammation levels in depressed adults with a history of childhood maltreatment. *Arch. Gen. Psychiatry* **2008**, *65*, 409–415. [CrossRef]
41. Vivar, C.; Potter, M.C.; van Praag, H. All about running: Synaptic plasticity, growth factors and adult hippocampal neurogenesis. *Curr. Top Behav. Neurosci.* **2013**, *15*, 189–210.
42. Ryan, S.M.; Nolan, Y.M. Neuroinflammation negatively affects adult hippocampal neurogenesis and cognition: Can exercise compensate? *Neurosci. Biobehav. Rev.* **2016**, *61*, 121–131. [CrossRef]
43. Song, H.; Peng, W.; Lee, K.M. Promoting exercise self-efficacy with an exergame. *J. Health Commun.* **2011**, *16*, 148–162. [CrossRef] [PubMed]
44. Viana, R.B.; de Lira, C.A.B. Exergames as coping strategies for anxiety disorders during the COVID-19 quarantine period. *Games Health* **2020**, *9*, 3. [CrossRef] [PubMed]
45. Wang, F.; Szabo, A. Effects of yoga on stress among healthy adults: A systematic review. *Altern. Ther. Health Med.* **2020**, *26*, AT6214.
46. Pellegrini, B.; Peyré-Tartaruga, L.; Zoppirolli, C.; Bortolan, L.; Bacchi, E.; Figard-Fabre, H.; Schena, F. Exploring muscle activation during nordic walking: A comparison between conventional and uphill walking. *PLoS ONE* **2015**, *10*, e0138906. [CrossRef] [PubMed]

47. Musumeci, G.; Carnazza, M.L.; Loreto, C.; Leonardi, R.; Loreto, C. β-Defensin-4 (HBD-4) is expressed in chondrocytes derived from normal and osteoarthritic cartilage encapsulated in PEGDA scaffold. *Acta Histochem.* **2012**, *114*, 805–812. [CrossRef] [PubMed]
48. Bieler, T.; Siersma, V.; Magnusson, S.P.; Kjaer, M.; Christensen, H.E.; Beyer, N. In hip osteoarthritis, Nordic Walking is superior to strength training and home-based exercise for improving function. *Scand. J. Med. Sci. Sports* **2017**, *27*, 873–886. [CrossRef] [PubMed]
49. Lipowski, M.; Walczak-Kozłowska, T.; Lipowska, M.; Kortas, J.; Antosiewicz, J.; Falcioni, G.; Ziemann, E. Improvement of attention, executive functions, and processing speed in elderly women as a result of involvement in the nordic walking training program and vitamin d supplementation. *Nutrients* **2019**, *11*, 1311. [CrossRef]
50. Park, S.D.; Yu, S.H. The effects of Nordic and general walking on depression disorder patients' depression, sleep, and body composition. *J. Phys. Ther. Sci.* **2015**, *27*, 2481–2485. [CrossRef]

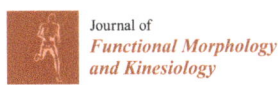

Journal of
Functional Morphology and Kinesiology

Article

Prevalence of Low Energy Availability in Collegiate Women Soccer Athletes

Meghan K. Magee [1,2], Brittanie L. Lockard [2,3], Hannah A. Zabriskie [4], Alexis Q. Schaefer [5], Joel A. Luedke [5], Jacob L. Erickson [6], Margaret T. Jones [1,2,*] and Andrew R. Jagim [2,5,6]

1. School of Kinesiology, George Mason University, Manassas, VA 20109, USA; mmagee2@gmu.edu
2. Patriot Performance Laboratory, Frank Pettrone Center for Sports Performance, Intercollegiate Athletics, George Mason University, Fairfax, VA 22030, USA; blockard@gmu.edu (B.L.L.); jagim.andrew@mayo.edu (A.R.J.)
3. Division of Human Performance, University of the Incarnate Word, San Antonio, TX 78209, USA
4. Department of Kinesiology, Towson University, Towson, MD 21252 USA; hzabriskie@towson.edu
5. Athletics Department, University of Wisconsin—La Crosse, La Crosse, WI 54601, USA; aschaefer@uwlax.edu (A.Q.S.); jluedke@uwlax.edu (J.A.L.)
6. Sports Medicine, Mayo Clinic Health System, Onalaska, WI 54650, USA; erickson.jacob@mayo.edu
* Correspondence: mjones15@gmu.edu

Received: 17 November 2020; Accepted: 16 December 2020; Published: 18 December 2020

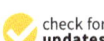

Abstract: (1) **Background:** Limited information exists on the prevalence of low energy availability (LEA) in collegiate team sports. The purpose of this study was to examine the prevalence of LEA in collegiate women soccer players. (2) **Methods:** Collegiate women soccer athletes ($n = 18$, height: 1.67 ± 0.05 m; body mass: 65.3 ± 7.9 kg; body fat %: $24.9 \pm 5.6\%$) had their body composition and sport nutrition knowledge assessed in the pre-season. Energy availability was assessed mid-season using a 4-day dietary log and activity energy expenditure values from a team-based monitoring system. A validated screening tool was used to screen for LEA. (3) **Results:** The screening tool classified 56.3% of athletes as at risk of LEA (<30 kcal/kg of FFM); however, the actual dietary intake identified 67% as LEA. Athletes identified as non-LEA consumed significantly more absolute ($p = 0.040$) and relative ($p = 0.004$) energy than LEA athletes. (4) **Conclusions:** There was a high prevalence of LEA among collegiate women soccer athletes. Although previously validated in women endurance athletes, the LEA screening tool was not effective in identifying those at risk of LEA in this sample of athletes.

Keywords: energy availability; relative energy deficiency in sport; sports nutrition; women soccer athletes; nutrition knowledge; LEAF-Q

---

1. Introduction

Athletes have specific dietary requirements in order to meet training demands and optimize performance [1]. Typically, athletes have higher activity levels; greater lean body mass; and require higher amounts of energy, protein, and carbohydrates per day compared to non-athletes. However, previous research has indicated that athletes often do not meet the nutritional guidelines specific to their level of training, with women athletes tending to exhibit dietary deficiencies more frequently than male athletes [2–12]. Insufficient energy intake may predispose an athlete to low energy availability (LEA), which is thought to be a primary contributor to a complex condition characterized by a multifactorial state of physiological dysfunction referred to as Relative Energy Deficiency in Sport (RED-S) syndrome [13]. The International Olympic Committee published a consensus statement on RED-S [13] which described RED-S as similar to the well-known Female Athlete Triad paradigm, but encompassing a broader definition to include a spectrum of physiological dysfunction attributable to chronic energy deficiency. This deficiency may result from insufficient energy intake, excessive energy expenditure from training, or a combination of both. Further, RED-S is commonly associated with reductions in performance, with a concomitant increased risk of health complications including, but not limited to, impairments in metabolism, menstrual function, bone health, immunity, protein synthesis, reproduction abilities, and cardiovascular health [13].

A common strategy to determine an athlete's risk of energy deficiency is to assess energy availability level (kcal/kg FFM/day), which is calculated by subtracting the activity energy expenditure from energy intake. Calculated energy availability values are commonly interpreted as follows: low < 30 kcal/kg FFM/day; moderate 30–45 kcal/kg FFM/day; optimal > 45 kcal/kg FFM/day (Ref. [14]). Energy availability serves as a means to quantify the residual energy available to support an athlete's physiological functions, and, if below a certain threshold, may be a primary causative factor contributing to RED-S over time [13]. Further, a higher prevalence of LEA is reported in women athletes, as indicated in previous studies [15–18]. Although valuable, the calculation of energy availability is laborious and can be challenging when working with a large number of athletes. Therefore, screening tools such as the Low Energy Availability in Females Questionnaire (LEAF-Q) [19] have been developed and previously validated in a cohort of women endurance athletes and dancers, but not collegiate team sport athletes. Certain body composition parameters, densitometry metrics, hematological markers, and metabolic tests have also been used to screen for those at risk of RED-S with variable degrees of efficacy [20–22]. A better understanding of the utility of these screening tools across multiple populations would help practitioners to identify athletes at risk of LEA.

Common trends among athletes regarding dietary practices indicate a misunderstanding of energy and macronutrient requirements and the role of certain dietary supplements [23], which likely contributes to the dietary deficiencies and occurrence of LEA commonly seen in athletes [24]. However, inconsistencies exist as to how the nutrition knowledge of athletes has been assessed in the past [23]. Therefore, in an effort to create a more standardized method of assessing nutrition knowledge, Trakman et al. [25,26] developed an abridged nutrition knowledge questionnaire that is specific to the dietary requirements of athletes. In theory, a higher level of nutrition knowledge may positively influence an athlete's dietary behaviors, as previous research in athletes has indicated that those with greater sport nutrition knowledge scores were more likely to self-report healthier dietary practices [27]. Further, previous sport nutrition education interventions have led to marked improvements in nutrition knowledge [4], quality of diet [4,28], body composition, and performance [28] over the course of a season. However, the potential relationship between nutrition knowledge and LEA in athletes has yet to be fully elucidated.

In the United States, Division III athletes represent ~39% of the National Collegiate Athletic Association, which includes more than 440 Division III women's soccer programs. Limited data exist in regard to LEA prevalence in collegiate team sport athletes, specifically in women's soccer. Likewise, the effectiveness of screening tools, such as the LEAF-Q, in identifying those at risk of LEA has yet to be determined, or how nutrition knowledge may influence energy availability in collegiate team sport athletes. Therefore, the purpose of the current study was to examine the prevalence of LEA among a convenience sample of Division III collegiate women soccer athletes and to examine the utility of the LEAF-Q as a tool to screen for those at risk of LEA. A secondary aim was to examine the relationship between nutrition knowledge, energy availability, and dietary intake.

2. Materials and Methods

2.1. Experimental Design

The current observational study began prior to the start of the fall academic term and soccer season, when athletes completed a body composition assessment and an electronic online survey previously developed to assess sport nutrition knowledge. At the soccer season's midpoint, athletes completed a different online electronic survey to screen for LEA. At this time, athletes also completed a 4-day monitoring period to assess energy availability. Players were asked to record dietary intake and were equipped with a team-based heart rate monitoring system with on-board inertial sensors to assess activity energy expenditure throughout each practice and match during the 4-day monitoring period.

2.2. Subjects

Eighteen National Collegiate Athletic Association (NCAA) Division III women soccer athletes participated in the current study. The participant demographic data are presented in Table 1. All players who were medically cleared were invited to participate in this study. Procedures were approved by the University's Institutional Review Board for the Protection of Human Subjects (IRB #19-AJ-707). The study was conducted according to the Declaration of Helsinki guidelines. Written consent was obtained from all the subjects prior to data collection.

Table 1. Summary of subject demographics ($n = 18$).

Height (m)	1.67 ± 0.1
Body Mass (kg)	65.3 ± 7.9
Fat Free Mass (kg)	49.1 ± 4.7
Body Fat (%)	24.9 ± 5.6
Age (yrs.)	19.2 ± 1.1

Values represented as mean ± standard deviation.

2.3. Procedures

Upon arrival to the laboratory, height and body mass were recorded to the nearest 0.01 cm and 0.02 kg, respectively, using a stadiometer (Detecto, Webb City, MO, USA) and digital scale (BOD POD model 2000A; BOD POD; Cosmed USA, Concord, CA, USA), with each subject barefoot. Body composition variables (i.e., percent body fat, fat-free mass, and fat mass) were assessed using air displacement plethysmography (BOD POD model 2000A; BOD POD; Cosmed USA, Concord, CA, USA) according to standard operating procedures. The thoracic gas volume was estimated.

2.3.1. Energy Availability

Athletes were asked to record dietary intake using an online commercially available nutrition analysis program (MyFitnessPal, Under Armour, Baltimore, MD, USA). Prior to this period, they were educated on methods to estimate portion sizes and provided with informational packets and instructional videos to promote accurate self-reporting. Daily energy and macronutrient intakes were averaged across the 4-day monitoring period. Absolute energy and macronutrient intakes (kcal/day or g/day) were recorded and were also made relative to body weight (kcal/kg/day or g/kg/day) to allow for comparison between individuals. Activity energy expenditure was assessed using wearable monitoring devices (Polar TeamPro™ Polar Electro, Oy, Finland) and calculated using proprietary algorithms. Energy availability was then calculated by subtracting the activity energy expenditure from energy intake and expressed as kcals per kilogram of FFM. A threshold of <30 kcal/kg of FFM was used to classify players as having LEA [14].

2.3.2. Low Energy Availability in Females Questionnaire

The LEAF-Q, originally developed as a paper survey, was converted into an online electronic format for ease of distribution and scoring. The 25-item questionnaire asks a series of questions pertaining to prior injury history, gastrointestinal issues, menstrual cycle patterns, and contraception use. A score of ≥8 would classify the athlete as having LEA. It has previously been shown to have an acceptable degree of sensitivity (78%) and specificity (90%) in women athletes and a Cronbach's alpha ≥ 0.71 [19].

2.3.3. Abridged Sport Nutrition Knowledge Questionnaire

The Abridged Sport Nutrition Knowledge Questionnaire (ANSKQ) consists of 37 items that assess general ($n = 17$) and sport ($n = 20$) nutrition knowledge and has previously been shown to be a valid and reliable questionnaire and has a PerSepIndex = 0.80 [29]. The scores from the ANSKQ were automatically calculated and categorized using the knowledge scoring system of poor (0–49%), average (50–65%), good (66–75%), and excellent (75–100%) from previously published methods [26].

3. Statistical Analysis

A sensitivity and specificity analysis was completed to examine the ability of the LEAF-Q to identify those at risk of LEA. Tests of normality were conducted, and it was found that Shapiro–Wilk was violated for average energy availability (AEA) for non-LEA athletes ($p = 0.044$) and for average energy intake (AEI) for LEA athletes. Thus, differences in AEA and AEI were assessed using the Mann–Whitney U test. Differences in other variables of energy intake between athletes having LEA and athletes without LEA were analyzed using independent samples t-tests. Data were considered statistically significant when the probability of a type I error was 0.05 or less. Pearson correlation coefficients were used to examine the relationships between EA, LEAF-Q scores, ASNKQ scores, BF %, FFM, fat mass, body mass, and body mass index. The following criteria were used for interpreting the correlation coefficients: very weak: <0.20; weak: 0.20–0.39; moderate: 0.40–0.59; strong: 0.60–0.79; and very strong: >0.80 [30]. Cohen's d, utilizing pooled standard deviations, was used to assess the effect sizes for differences in the energy intake variables. The effect sizes were interpreted using the following criteria: 0.2 = trivial; 0.2–0.6 = small; 0.7–1.2 = moderate; 1.3–2.0 = large; and >2.0 = very large. All the data were analyzed using the Statistical Package for the Social Sciences (SPSS, Version 25.0; IBM Corp., Armonk, NY, USA).

4. Results

A total of 66.7% percent of athletes ($n = 12$) presented with LEA (23.0 ± 5.7 kcals/kg FFM) versus non-LEA ($n = 6$; 36.4 ± 7.3 kcals/kg FFM). The LEAF-Q survey tool only identified 56.3% of athletes as at risk of LEA. The sensitivity and specificity analysis yielded a true positive rate of 40.0% and a true negative rate of 16.7% when using the LEAF-Q as a screening tool for LEA.

Table 2 provides a summary of the dietary intake of all athletes. In comparison to athletes with LEA, athletes without LEA consumed more relative ($p = 0.004$) energy than those with LEA. Athletes without LEA also consumed higher amounts of carbohydrates (absolute: $p = 0.029$; relative: $p = 0.003$) and relative fat ($p = 0.013$) than LEA athletes. No differences were observed between the absolute and relative protein consumed or the absolute fat intake. Additionally, there were no differences in the absolute energy intake between the two groups.

The mean score from the ASNKQ indicated that 44.7% of the questions were answered correctly. When analyzing the difference in scores between the athletes with and without LEA, the athletes with LEA scored lower compared to the athletes without LEA (40.9 ± 10.4% vs. 52.4 ± 9.8%; $p = 0.040$; ES = 1.14). Moderate inverse relationships were observed between the mean energy availability values and body mass ($r = -0.503$) and FFM ($r = -0.520$), and between the ASNKQ scores and fat mass ($r = -0.508$), as presented in Table 3.

Table 2. A summary of average daily energy and macronutrient intake by energy status.

	LEA (*n* = 12)	Non-LEA (*n* = 6)	All (*n* = 18)	Effect Size
Energy Availability (kcals/kg FFM/d)	23.0 ± 5.7	36.4 ± 7.3	27.5 ± 8.9	2.0
Energy Intake (kcal/d)	1806.8 ± 264.0	2179.7 ± 452.0 *	1931.2 ± 371.2	1.0
Relative Energy Intake (kcals/kg/d)	26.9 ± 5.2	36.5 ± 7.0 **	30.1 ± 7.3	1.6
Carbohydrate Intake (g/d)	220.1 ± 36.6	274.3 ± 59.8 *	238.2 ± 51.1	1.1
Relative Carbohydrate intake (g/kg/d)	3.3 ± 0.7	4.6 ± 0.9 **	3.7 ± 1.0	1.6
Protein Intake (g/d)	74.5 ± 17.0	81.1 ± 22.3	76.7 ± 18.5	0.3
Relative Protein Intake (g/kg/d)	1.1 ± 0.3	1.3 ± 0.3	1.2 ± 0.3	0.7
Fat Intake (g/d)	64.1 ± 12.	82.7 ± 26.7	70.3 ± 19.6	0.9
Relative Fat Intake (g/kg/d)	1.0 ± 0.2	1.4 ± 0.4 *	1.1 ± 0.4	1.3

Values represented as mean ± standard deviation. * $p < 0.05$, ** $p < 0.01$.

Table 3. Relationships between body composition parameters, energy availability, and sport nutrition knowledge.

	Body Mass (kg)	BF% (%)	FFM (kg)	FM (kg)	Mean EA (kcal/kg FFM)	LEAFQ Score (AU)	ASNKQ (% Correct)
Body Mass (kg)	1	0.479 *	0.774 **	0.828 **	−0.503 *	−0.068	−0.322
BF% (%)		1	−0.135	0.771 **	−0.068	−0.116	−0.183
FFM (kg)			1	0.301	−0.520 *	0.014	−0.066
FM (kg)				1	−0.324	−0.116	−0.508 *
Mean EA (kcal/kg FFM)					1	0.088	0.117
LEAFQ Score (AU)						1	0.410
ASNKQ (% Correct)							1

* Correlation is significant at the 0.05 level (2-tailed). ** Correlation is significant at the 0.01 level (2-tailed). BF% = body fat percentage; FFM = fat-free mass; FM = fat mass; EA = energy availability; LEAFQ = low energy availability in females questionnaire; ASNKQ = abridged sport nutrition knowledge questionnaire.

5. Discussion

The purpose of the current study was to assess the prevalence of LEA among a cohort of collegiate women soccer athletes and to examine the utility of the LEAF-Q as a tool to screen for those at risk of LEA. A secondary aim was to assess the relationship between nutrition knowledge, energy availability, and energy intake. The main findings of the current study found the prevalence of LEA to be 67% among the current cohort of athletes when assessed directly through dietary analysis and activity energy expenditure. This prevalence rate is higher than previous findings reported in women soccer players at the NCAA Division I (26–33%) [31] and professional levels (23%) [32], as well as in collegiate volleyball (20%) [33] and elite endurance athletes (12–20%) [19]. However, prevalence rates of 40–60% have been observed in collegiate women endurance athletes [15,16], which are only slightly below those observed in the current study. Such similarity was unexpected, considering that, unlike soccer, success in endurance sports requires a high training volume and typically a smaller body type with minimal body fat, which predisposes one to LEA. Therefore, it would be expected that soccer athletes would be less likely to exhibit LEA compared to endurance athletes. The mean energy availability value observed in the current study was 27.5 ± 8.9 kcals/kg FFM/day, which is below the threshold of <30 kcals/kg FFM/day used to classify those with LEA [14], and below that previously reported in women soccer athletes at the professional level (35 kcals/kg FFM/day) [32]. Further, the aforementioned professional soccer athletes [32] had access to nutritional staff, compared to athletes in the current study whose institution did not staff a sport dietitian or nutritionist.

The high degree of variability in the LEA values across different team sports may be partially attributed to the limited access to sports nutrition education and provisional food (fueling stations), resources that may be more common at more competitive collegiate and elite levels. In fact, previous research has indicated that sport nutrition education interventions and access to a sports dietitian improve eating behaviors and nutritional knowledge in collegiate athletes [4,34,35]. However, some studies have shown [15,36] that, while a nutritional education intervention led to a measurable increase in nutrition knowledge, the prevalence of LEA did not change. Therefore, a combined approach of nutrition education, opportunities to practice dietary skills as well as behavior change therapy [37] may be necessary to help athletes minimize the risk of nutritional deficiencies [38].

The results from the current study indicate that the LEAF-Q was not an effective screening tool, as it only identified 56.3% of the soccer athletes as at risk of LEA, while the direct assessment of LEA identified 66.7% of the athletes as exhibiting LEA. Further, the sensitivity and specificity analysis yielded significantly lower values than those previously published when the tool was validated [19]. Similar findings have also been reported at the professional level [32]; therefore, the LEAF-Q may have limited utility as a screening instrument in women's soccer, at least when used as a standalone tool. The LEAF-Q has been used successfully in elite sprinters for identifying LEA in conjunction with additional primary indicators, including energy availability, the presence of amenorrhea, low bone mineral density, and hormone abnormalities [39]. Therefore, a comprehensive monitoring plan may be warranted in order to accurately screen athletes and those at risk or in need of further clinical evaluations.

A novel finding from the current study was that athletes with LEA scored lower (41% = poor) on the ANSKQ than athletes without LEA (52% = average) [26], suggesting that lower nutrition knowledge may increase the likelihood of insufficient energy intake, as athletes may have less of an understanding of how to meet the dietary requirements of their sport. Further, moderate differences between those with LEA and those without, as determined by effect size, were observed. Additionally, an inverse relationship was observed between nutrition knowledge and fat mass ($r = -0.508$), indicating that athletes with lower nutrition knowledge had higher levels of fat mass. There were no additional relationships between nutrition knowledge, energy availability, and body composition values.

Low energy availability values are one of many metrics that may indicate dietary insufficiencies. The athletes in the current study had a daily mean energy intake of 30 kcals/kg/day, which is below the recommended energy intake of 40–60 kcals/kg for women team sport athletes [7,40] and likely contributed to the high prevalence of LEA observed. Similar findings have been reported in the Under−21 United States Women's National Soccer team, with an average daily energy intake of 34 kcals/kg/day reported [8]. Additionally, the daily carbohydrate intake of 3.7 g/kg per day observed in the current study was below the recommended 5–12 g/kg of bodyweight for soccer players [41]. This finding is consistent with other studies in women's soccer, which have frequently noted inadequate carbohydrate intakes ranging from 3.3 to 5.0 g/kg/day [8–12,32]. In the current study, suboptimal energy and macronutrient intakes were more common in athletes with LEA (Table 2). The inability of collegiate athletes to meet nutritional recommendations for their respective sport is not uncommon, as it has been previously reported in both men and women athletes participating in football [42], lacrosse [7], swimming [6], basketball [2], gymnastics [2], and volleyball [33]. While nutritional recommendations have been established for women soccer athletes, the results of the current study demonstrate a continued need for sport nutrition education interventions to be part of regular team activities. Moreover, the high prevalence of LEA is concerning and supports the need to identify individuals at risk of LEA, particularly at lower levels of competition, who may not have access to sport dietitians or other nutrition-centric resources. The early detection of LEA and the implementation of appropriate interventions may reduce the risk of conditions such as RED-S. Therefore, there remains a need for accurate and efficient screening tools to identify those at risk of LEA.

6. Limitations

A limitation of the current study is the use of self-reported dietary intake, which may be subject to underreporting by participants [43]. Therefore, there is a potential bias for an overestimation in the prevalence of LEA. Further, the 4-day monitoring period may not be an adequate reflection of the normal dietary habits and activity levels of the athletes throughout the entire season. Therefore, it is possible that, while the LEAF-Q did not accurately identify those at risk of LEA when compared to direct measures of energy availability, the LEAF-Q may be more reflective of long-term energy status, as the questions are directed at health history and symptoms common to RED-S, which may manifest over time. An additional limitation is the small sample size. The prevalence of LEA among the current cohort of women soccer athletes may not be representative of all women soccer athletes across all levels of collegiate competition.

7. Conclusions

The results indicate there may be a high prevalence of LEA among collegiate women soccer athletes. Since the LEAF-Q was not an effective tool in identifying those at risk of LEA, it is recommended that future research examine the utility of LEAF-Q for women athletes participating in team sports. Additionally, the nutrition knowledge of collegiate women soccer athletes was classified as poor-to-average, with the athletes failing to meet several nutritional recommendations for their respective level of training. Athletes with LEA tended to have a lower nutrition knowledge score compared to those without LEA. Therefore, the development of additional screening tools for LEA would be beneficial for the team sport population. Sport nutrition education interventions are recommended to help athletes understand their advanced dietary requirements and provide practical strategies to meet these dietary recommendations. This may help athletes consume adequate amounts of energy and avoid having LEA.

Author Contributions: Conceptualization, A.R.J., J.A.L. and J.L.E.; methodology, A.R.J., A.Q.S. and J.A.L.; software, A.R.J., A.Q.S. and J.A.L.; formal analysis, A.R.J. and H.A.Z.; investigation, A.R.J., A.Q.S. and J.A.L.; resources, A.R.J., J.A.L. and J.L.E.; data curation, A.R.J., H.A.Z. and A.Q.S.; writing—original draft preparation, A.R.J., M.K.M., B.L.L. and M.T.J.; writing—review and editing, M.K.M., B.L.L., H.A.Z., J.L.E., M.T.J. and A.R.J.; visualization, A.R.J.; supervision, A.Q.S., J.A.L., J.L.E. and A.R.J. All authors have read and agreed to the published version of the manuscript.

Funding: This research received no external funding.

Acknowledgments: The authors would like to thank all the women soccer players and coaching staff who participated in this project and supported the study procedures.

Conflicts of Interest: The authors declare no conflict of interest.

References

1. American Dietetic Association; Dietitians of Canada; American College of Sports Medicine; Rodriguez, N.R.; Di Marco, N.M.; Langley, S. American College of Sports Medicine position stand. Nutrition and athletic performance. *Med. Sci. Sports Exerc.* **2009**, *41*, 709–731. [CrossRef] [PubMed]
2. Hickson, J.F., Jr.; Schrader, J.; Trischler, L.C. Dietary intakes of female basketball and gymnastics athletes. *J. Am. Diet. Assoc.* **1986**, *86*, 251–253. [PubMed]
3. Hinton, P.S.; Sanford, T.C.; Davidson, M.M.; Yakushko, O.F.; Beck, N.C. Nutrient intakes and dietary behaviors of male and female collegiate athletes. *Int. J. Sport Nutr. Exerc. Metab.* **2004**, *14*, 389–405. [CrossRef] [PubMed]
4. Valliant, M.W.; Emplaincourt, H.P.; Wenzel, R.K.; Garner, B.H. Nutrition education by a registered dietitian improves dietary intake and nutrition knowledge of a NCAA female volleyball team. *Nutrients* **2012**, *4*, 506–516. [CrossRef]
5. Beals, K.A. Eating behaviors, nutritional status, and menstrual function in elite female adolescent volleyball players. *J. Am. Diet. Assoc.* **2002**, *102*, 1293–1296. [CrossRef]
6. Hoogenboom, B.J.; Morris, J.; Morris, C.; Schaefer, K. Nutritional knowledge and eating behaviors of female, collegiate swimmers. *NAJSPT* **2009**, *4*, 139–148.
7. Jagim, A.; Zabriskie, H.; Currier, B.; Harty, P.; Stecker, R.; Kerksick, C. Nutrient status and perceptions of energy and macronutrient intake in a group of collegiate female lacrosse athletes. *J. Int. Soc. Sports Nutr.* **2019**, *16*, 43. [CrossRef]

8. Mullinix, M.C.; Jonnalagadda, S.S.; Rosenbloom, C.A.; Thompson, W.R.; Kicklighter, J.R. Dietary intake of female US soccer players. *Nutr. Res.* **2003**, *23*, 585–593. [CrossRef]
9. Martin, L.; Lambeth, A.; Scott, D. Nutritional practices of national female soccer players: Analysis and recommendations. *J. Sports Sci. Med.* **2006**, *5*, 130–137.
10. Clark, M.; Reed, D.B.; Crouse, S.F.; Armstrong, R.B. Pre- and post-season dietary intake, body composition, and performance indices of NCAA division I female soccer players. *Int. J. Sport Nutr. Exerc. Metab.* **2003**, *13*, 303–319. [CrossRef]
11. Gibson, J.C.; Stuart-Hill, L.; Martin, S.; Gaul, C. Nutrition status of junior elite Canadian female soccer athletes. *Int. J. Soc. Sports Nutr.* **2011**, *21*, 507–514. [CrossRef] [PubMed]
12. Dobrowolski, H.; Wlodarek, D. Low energy availability in group of Polish female soccer players. *Rocz. Panstw. Zakl. Hig.* **2020**, *71*, 89–96. [CrossRef]
13. Mountjoy, M.; Sundgot-Borgen, J.K.; Burke, L.M.; Ackerman, K.E.; Blauwet, C.; Constantini, N.; Lebrun, C.; Lundy, B.; Melin, A.K.; Meyer, N.L.; et al. IOC consensus statement on relative energy deficiency in sport (RED-S): 2018 update. *Br. J. Sports Med.* **2018**, *52*, 687–697. [CrossRef] [PubMed]
14. Loucks, A.B.; Kiens, B.; Wright, H.H. Energy availability in athletes. *J. Sports Sci.* **2011**, *29* (Suppl. 1), S7–S15. [CrossRef] [PubMed]
15. Day, J.; Wengreen, H.; Heath, E.; Brown, K. Prevalence of low energy availability in collegiate female runners and implementation of nutrition education intervention. *Sports Nutr. Ther.* **2015**, *1*, 1. [CrossRef]
16. Beermann, B.L.; Lee, D.G.; Almstedt, H.C.; McCormack, W.P. Nutritional intake and energy availability of collegiate distance runners. *J. Am. Coll. Nutr.* **2020**, 1–9. [CrossRef]
17. Viner, R.T.; Harris, M.; Berning, J.R.; Meyer, N.L. Energy Availability and Dietary Patterns of Adult Male and female competitive cyclists with lower than expected bone mineral density. *Int. J. Sports Nutr. Exerc. Metab.* **2015**, *25*, 594–602. [CrossRef]
18. Doyle-Lucas, A.F.; Akers, J.D.; Davy, B.M. Energetic efficiency, menstrual irregularity, and bone mineral density in elite professional female ballet dancers. *J. Dance Med. Sci.* **2010**, *14*, 146–154.
19. Melin, A.; Tornberg, A.B.; Skouby, S.; Faber, J.; Ritz, C.; Sjodin, A.; Sundgot-Borgen, J. The LEAF questionnaire: A screening tool for the identification of female athletes at risk for the female athlete triad. *Br. J. Sports Med.* **2014**, *48*, 540–545. [CrossRef]
20. Melin, A.K.; Heikura, I.A.; Tenforde, A.; Mountjoy, M. Energy availability in athletics: Health, performance, and physique. *Int. J. Sports Nutr. Exerc. Metab.* **2019**, *29*, 152–164. [CrossRef]
21. Staal, S.; Sjodin, A.; Fahrenholtz, I.; Bonnesen, K.; Melin, A.K. Low RMR ratio as a surrogate marker for energy deficiency, the choice of predictive equation vital for correctly identifying male and female ballet dancers at risk. *Int. J. Sports Nutr. Exec. Metab.* **2018**, *28*, 412–418. [CrossRef] [PubMed]
22. Heikura, I.A.; Uusitalo, A.L.T.; Stellingwerff, T.; Bergland, D.; Mero, A.A.; Burke, L.M. Low energy availability is difficult to assess but outcomes have large impact on bone injury rates in elite distance athletes. *Int. J. Sports Nutr. Exec. Metab.* **2018**, *28*, 403–411. [CrossRef] [PubMed]
23. Trakman, G.L.; Forsyth, A.; Devlin, B.L.; Belski, R. A systematic review of athletes' and coaches' nutrition knowledge and reflections on the quality of current nutrition knowledge measures. *Nutrients* **2016**, *8*, 570. [CrossRef] [PubMed]
24. Areta, J.L.; Taylor, H.L.; Koehler, K. Low energy availability: History, definition and evidence of its endocrine, metabolic and physiological effects in prospective studies in females and males. *Eur. J. Appl. Physiol.* **2020**. [CrossRef] [PubMed]
25. Trakman, G.L.; Brown, F.; Forsyth, A.; Belski, R. Modifications to the nutrition for sport knowledge questionnaire (NSQK) and abridged nutrition for sport knowledge questionnaire (ANSKQ). *J. Int. Soc. Sports Nutr.* **2019**, *16*, 26. [CrossRef]
26. Trakman, G.L.; Forsyth, A.; Hoye, R.; Belski, R. The nutrition for sport knowledge questionnaire (NSKQ): Development and validation using classical test theory and Rasch analysis. *J. Int. Soc. Sports Nutr.* **2017**, *14*, 26. [CrossRef]
27. Alaunyte, I.; Perry, J.L.; Aubrey, T. Nutritional knowledge and eating habits of professional rugby league players: Does knowledge translate into practice? *J. Int. Soc. Sports Nutr.* **2015**, *12*, 18. [CrossRef]
28. Rossi, F.E.; Landreth, A.; Beam, S.; Jones, T.; Norton, L.; Cholewa, J.M. The effects of a sports nutrition education intervention on nutritional status, sport nutrition knowledge, body composition, and performance during off season training in NCAA Division I baseball players. *J. Sports Sci. Med.* **2017**, *16*, 60–68.

29. Trakman, G.L.; Forsyth, A.; Hoye, R.; Belski, R. Development and validation of a brief general and sports nutrition knowledge questionnaire and assessment of athletes' nutrition knowledge. *J. Int. Soc. Sports Nutr.* **2018**, *15*, 17. [CrossRef]
30. Evans, J.D. *Straightforward Statistics for the Behavioral Sciences*; Thomson Brooks/Cole Publishing Co.: Pacific Grove, CA, USA, 1996.
31. Reed, J.L.; De Souza, M.J.; Williams, N.I. Changes in energy availability across the season in Division I female soccer players. *J. Sports Sci.* **2013**, *31*, 314–324. [CrossRef]
32. Moss, S.L.; Randell, R.K.; Burgess, D.; Ridley, S.; ÓCairealláin, C.; Allison, R.; Rollo, I. Assessment of energy availability and associated risk factors in professional female soccer players. *Eur. J. Sport Sci.* **2020**, 1–10. [CrossRef] [PubMed]
33. Woodruff, S.J.; Meloche, R.D. Energy availability of female varsity volleyball players. *Int. J. Sports Nutr. Exec. Metab.* **2013**, *23*, 24–30. [CrossRef] [PubMed]
34. Hull, M.V.; Jagim, A.R.; Oliver, J.M.; Greenwood, M.; Busteed, D.R.; Jones, M.T. Gender differences and access to a sports dietitian influence dietary habits of collegiate athletes. *J. Int. Soc. Sports Nutr.* **2016**, *13*, 38. [CrossRef] [PubMed]
35. Hull, M.V.; Neddo, J.; Jagim, A.R.; Oliver, J.M.; Greenwood, M.; Jones, M.T. Availability of a sports dietitian may lead to improved performance and recovery of NCAA division I baseball athletes. *J. Int. Soc. Sports Nutr.* **2017**, *14*, 29. [CrossRef]
36. Zawila, L.G.; Steib, C.S.; Hoogenboom, B. The female collegiate cross-country runner: Nutritional knowledge and attitudes. *J. Athl. Train* **2003**, *38*, 67–74.
37. Waldrop, J. Early identification and interventions for female athlete triad. *J. Pediatr. Health Care* **2005**, *19*, 213–220. [CrossRef]
38. Bentley, M.R.N.; Patterson, L.B.; Mitchell, N.; Backhouse, S.H. Athlete perspectives on the enablers and barriers to nutritional adherence in high-performing sport. *Psychol. Sports Exer.* **2020**, *52*, 101831. [CrossRef]
39. Sygo, J.; Coates, A.M.; Sesbreno, E.; Mountjoy, M.L.; Burr, J.F. Prevalence of indicators of low energy availability in elite female sprinters. *Int. J. Sports Nutr. Exec. Metab.* **2018**, *28*, 490–496. [CrossRef]
40. Kerksick, C.M.; Wilborn, C.D.; Roberts, M.D.; Smith-Ryan, A.; Kleiner, S.M.; Jager, R.; Collins, R.; Cooke, M.; Davis, J.N.; Galvan, E.; et al. ISSN exercise & sports nutrition review update: Research & recommendations. *J. Int. Soc. Sports Nutr.* **2018**, *15*, 38. [CrossRef]
41. Dobrowolski, H.; Karczemna, A.; Wlodarek, D. Nutrition for Female Soccer Players-Recommendations. *Medicina* **2020**, *56*, 28. [CrossRef]
42. Jagim, A.R.; Wright, G.A.; Kisiolek, J.; Jones, M.T.; Oliver, J.M. Position specific changes in body composition, hydration status, and metabolism during preseason training camp and nutritional habits of Division III football players. *Open Sport Sci. J.* **2016**, *10*, 17–26. [CrossRef]
43. Schoeller, D.A.; Bandini, L.G.; Dietz, W.H. Inaccuracies in self-reported intake identified by comparison with the doubly labelled water method. *Can. J. Physiol. Pharmacol.* **1990**, *68*, 941–949. [CrossRef] [PubMed]

Publisher's Note: MDPI stays neutral with regard to jurisdictional claims in published maps and institutional affiliations.

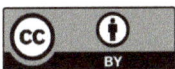

© 2020 by the authors. Licensee MDPI, Basel, Switzerland. This article is an open access article distributed under the terms and conditions of the Creative Commons Attribution (CC BY) license (http://creativecommons.org/licenses/by/4.0/).

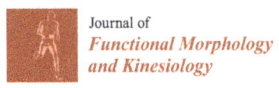

Journal of
Functional Morphology and Kinesiology

Article

Effects of Dehydration on Archery Performance, Subjective Feelings and Heart Rate during a Competition Simulation

Alexandros Savvides, Christoforos D. Giannaki, Angelos Vlahoyiannis, Pinelopi S. Stavrinou and George Aphamis *

Department of Life and Health Sciences, University of Nicosia, 46 Makedonitissas Avenue, CY1700 Nicosia, Cyprus; Savvides.A4@live.unic.ac.cy (A.S.); giannaki.c@unic.ac.cy (C.D.G.); vlahoyiannis.a@unic.ac.cy (A.V.); stavrinou.p@unic.ac.cy (P.S.S.)
* Correspondence: aphamis.g@unic.ac.cy

Received: 17 July 2020; Accepted: 25 August 2020; Published: 27 August 2020

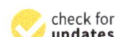

Abstract: This study aimed to investigate the effect of dehydration on archery performance, subjective feelings and heart rate response. Ten national level archers performed two archery competition simulations, once under euhydration (EUH) and once in a dehydrated state (DEH), induced by 24-h reduced fluid intake. Hydration status was verified prior to each trial by urine specific gravity (USG ≥ 1.025). Archery score was measured according to official archery regulations. Subjective feelings of thirst, fatigue and concentration were recorded on a visual analogue scale. Heart rate was continuously monitored during the trials. Archery performance was similar between trials ($p = 0.155$). During DEH trial (USG 1.032 ± 0.005), the athletes felt thirstier ($p < 0.001$), more fatigued ($p = 0.041$) and less able to concentrate ($p = 0.016$) compared with the EUH trial (USG 1.015 ± 0.004). Heart rate during DEH at baseline (85 ± 5 b·min^{-1}) was higher ($p = 0.021$) compared with EUH (78 ± 6 b·min^{-1}) and remained significantly higher during the latter stages of the DEH compared to EUH trial. In conclusion, archery performance over 72 arrows was not affected by dehydration, despite the induced psychological and physiological strain, revealed from decreased feeling of concentration, increased sensation of fatigue and increased heart rate during the DEH trial.

Keywords: hydration; urine specific gravity; athletes; heart rate; fatigue; alertness

---

1. Introduction

Hydration is of considerable interest for health, thermoregulation, as well as sports and athletic performance. A cascade of physiological responses even to a mild deficit in total body water hinders the body's ability to thermoregulate and maintain blood flow [1]. Decreased plasma volume leads to decreased blood flow to the exercising muscles and contributes further to impaired aerobic capacity [1,2] on various athletic disciplines such as cycling [2,3], long-distance running [4] and rowing [5]. Water losses and ensuing hyperthermia during exercise can also impair team sports or tennis performance [6] and muscular endurance [7] but not maximum strength or power [8].

Archery requires a repetitive motion with great precision, and therefore, its physiological demands are not similar to other predominately aerobic or anaerobic sports. During each arrow throw, one arm is used to hold (push) the bow in a steady position while the other arm pulls the bow string, with increasing muscle tremor in order to hold arrow-target alignment until the release of the arrow [9]. It has been estimated that the average force required to pull the bow is 20 kg for the men and 18 kg for the women. When this is multiplied by the number of arrow throws during a competition, one can get the total workload required by the exercising muscles in the shoulder area [10] and the trapezoid muscle [11].

This requires potentially a degree of muscular endurance over the duration of the competition, which could be affected by dehydration [7], especially under certain environmental conditions, as for example increased ambient temperature. Furthermore, archers must maintain a steady posture and body alignment with the target, in order to be as successful as possible. Even moderate intensity exercise combined with dehydration can lead to altered posture and increased muscle tremor, whereas euhydration allows for good muscle function and retention of postural control [12].

In archers, cardiovascular system also undergoes a specific stress during training [13] and competition [14]. Quality shooting for hours has been shown to challenge cardiovascular fitness and hand-eye coordination [15]. Increased ambient temperature could amplify the burden of inadequate hydration levels, which in turn may lead not only to reduced aerobic performance [1], but also to decreased brain volume [16] and altered brain function [17]. Dehydration can also negatively affect mood and vigilance [18,19], and increase tension, anxiety and fatigue [18], adding to the existing archers' competition stress.

So far, with regards to archery performance during competition, little is known about the effects of fluid restriction and dehydration on skill performance, cognitive function and especially hand-eye coordination, as well as subjective feelings of fatigue and concentration of archers. Notably, findings from a laboratory setting may differ from actual results in a real competition scenario, and thus, the primary aim of the present study was to investigate archery performance under a dehydration state, following 24 h of restricted fluid intake, during a simulated competition in a hot environment. Secondary aims were to monitor heart rate (HR) responses and subjective feelings related to dehydration (thirst, alertness, concentration, fatigue) during an archery competition simulation.

2. Materials and Methods

2.1. Participants

Ten national level archers (males $n = 7$, females $n = 3$; age: 22 ± 3 year, height 171 ± 9 cm, body mass 74.4 ± 11.9 kg) volunteered for this study. All participants were at the advanced level, training regularly 5–6 days per week, 2–3 h per day and competing for at least two years in Division A of the national championship. Any kind of history of major disease or medication was strictly considered as exclusion criterion. All athletes were informed for the purposes of the study and provided a written consent form. The study was approved by the Cyprus National Biothetics Committee on 5th July 2019 (Project ID: EEBK/EΠ/2018/13). All procedures were conducted according to the manual of the Declaration of Helsinki in 1964 and its later amendments.

2.2. Study Design

An overview of study design is depicted in Figure 1. Data collection took place during the competitive period at the Cyprus Archery Federation facilities. During this study, the temperature was 36–37 °C, and relative humidity was 81–83%. Participants visited the accredited archery area on two occasions, in counterbalanced order, once under euhydration (EUH) and once under a dehydrated state (DEH) induced by a 24-h controlled fluid intake. The two trials took place in the morning (warm up started at 8:20 a.m. and the last arrow throw was completed by 10:50 a.m.) 7 days apart. Upon arrival at the archery area, anthropometrics were measured and hydration levels were assessed. Participants underwent a warm-up, followed by the competition simulation. Heart rate was monitored through the trials. Self-perceived feelings were recorded at the start and end of each session.

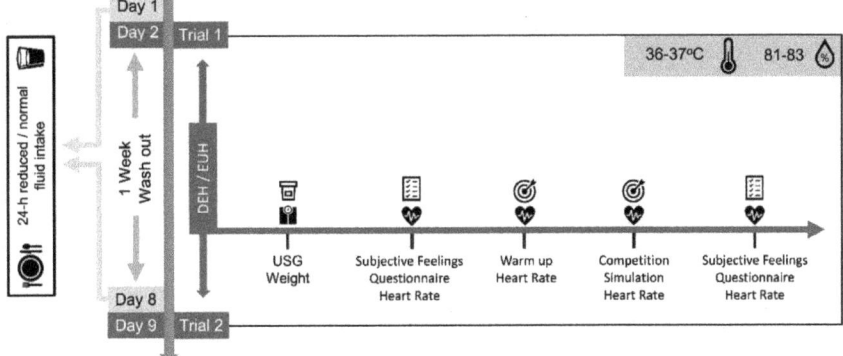

Figure 1. Overview of study design. DEH: Dehydration; EUH: Euhydration; USG: Urine Specific Gravity.

2.3. Fluid Restriction Protocol

All participants received dietary instructions to follow during all the study protocol, in order to avoid any nutrient deficiency. Caffeinated beverages, nutritional supplements and alcohol were not permitted for 48 h prior to trials. During the last 24 h prior to the trials, the participants followed the same isoenergetic nutritional plan, with a macronutrient distribution of 20%, 55% and 25% for protein, carbohydrate and fat, respectively. The nutrition plan was analyzed with Nutrilog Software v 2.60 (Marans, France), and the water content of the diet was approximately 1.2 L (0.9 L as water content of foods and 0.3 L as a result of macronutrient oxidation). In the dehydration scenario, the archers were further provided with 250 mL fluids at five intervals (total amount of fluids 5×250 mL = 1.25 L) during the last 24 h before the competition simulation. In the euhydration scenario, fluid intake was also standardized, providing archers with 500 mL fluids at breakfast, lunch and dinner and 250 mL of fluids at six intervals across the day (total amount of fluids $(3 \times 500$ mL$) + (6 \times 250$ mL$) = 3$ L).

2.4. Archery Competition Simulation Protocol

The competition simulation protocol consisted of a standardized warm-up, followed by the main archery competition phase. During the warm-up, each participant occupied one shooting line and upon a signal from the referee the participants shot 2 sets of 6 arrows at a 5-m distance targets over a 4-min period with a 3-min break between sets in order to collect the arrows. Then, the participants shot 2 rounds of 6 arrows at 70 m targets, again each round within a 4-min time frame, with 3 min break for arrow collection, and rested for 10 min before the main competition phase began.

During the competition phase, the archers assumed their position in their respective shooting lines and shot 6 rounds of 6 arrows. According to the regulations, 4 min were allowed for each round to be completed, followed by a 3-min break to collect arrows and write down the score for each participant. This was followed by a 10-min rest break, before continuing with another round of 6 arrows, until all 6 rounds were completed. The archery competition simulation was conducted according to the regulations of the International Archery Federation, at the Olympic distance of 70 m. All health and safety measures were taken according to the international competition rules. No food or fluid ingestion was allowed during the two main trials.

2.5. Anthropometrics

Upon arrival at the archery area, body mass (kg) was measured (participants wearing shorts and t-shirt only) using a portable scale (Seca model 755, Hamburg, Germany). Height (cm) was measured with a standing stadiometer (Seca model 720, Hamburg Germany).

2.6. Hydration Status Assessment

In the morning of each experimental trial, before study procedures, participants provided a first-morning-urine sample in a 60-mL container. Urine specific gravity (USG) was measured upon arrival of the participants at the archery center using a urine refractometer (DIGIT 0–12, Medline Scientific Limited, UK), to record hydration status. Euhydration/hypohydration cut-off point was set at USG < 1.025 [20]. All remaining urine was disposed down the toilet immediately after. No biological samples were stored after the determination of urine specific gravity.

2.7. Heart Rate Response

After urine collection, participants were allowed to rest, sitting comfortably, while a heart rate monitor (Polar H7, Polar Electro Oy, Professorintie S, FI-90440, Kempele, Finland) was attached on the participants' chest in order to continuously monitor heart rate throughout the exercise trials. Heart rate during the trials was recorded at baseline, end of the rest break after throw 6 and at the end of each throw.

2.8. Subjective Feelings Monitoring

At baseline and at the end of each trial, participants completed a subjective feelings questionnaire [21]. Athletes self-rated their feelings on thirst, fatigue, alertness and ability to concentrate on a 0–10 visual analogue scale, where "0" was "not-at-all" and "10" was "very much".

2.9. Statistical Analysis

Statistical analysis was performed with IBM®SPSS® statistics for Windows, version 25.0 (IBM Corp, Armonk, NY, USA). Data are reported as mean ± standard deviation. Differences on archery performance (total score) were detected with a paired-samples t-test. The normality of data was assessed by the Kolmogorov–Smirnov test. All data were normally distributed, and comparisons on subjective feelings between trials and over time (baseline vs. end of archery competition) were made with a two-way Repeated Measures ANOVA (time point × trial). Heart rate response at rest and after arrow throw was also analyzed with two-way Repeated Measures ANOVA (time point × trial). Bonferroni post-hoc analysis was performed where necessary. Effect sizes were calculated using partial eta squared (η^2) interpreted as 0.01 for small, 0.06 for moderate and 0.14 for large. Statistical significance was set at $p < 0.05$. Statistical power analysis was performed using the G*Power 3.1 power analysis software. Post hoc power analysis revealed that the sample size of the present study was adequate to provide statistical power of both heart rate and other main parameters of the study such as fatigue, concentration and thirst) with >90% power and with a significance level, $\alpha = 0.05$.

3. Results

Measurements of USG at baseline showed that USG at the DEH trial was 1.032 ± 0.005, which was above the dehydration cut off level for all athletes, and it was also higher ($p < 0.001$) than USG at the EUH trial (1.015 ± 0.004). This confirms that the participants performed the archery competition under the desired hydration state at each trial.

Total archery score was not different between trials (EUH 550 ± 63 points vs. DEH 562 ± 59 points; ($p = 0.155$)). No significant correlation was found between archery performance and USG levels (Figure 2).

Subjective feelings analysis (Figure 3) showed different responses between conditions. Regarding thirst, there was a trial effect ($F_{1,9} = 45.6$, $p < 0.001$, $\eta^2 = 0.836$), a time effect ($F_{1,9} = 56.5$, $p < 0.001$, $\eta^2 = 0.863$) and a time × time interaction ($F_{1,9} = 10.5$, $p = 0.010$, $\eta^2 = 0.538$), as sensation of thirst was higher at baseline of the DEH trial compared with EUH ($p = 0.003$) and thirst increased over time during both trials (EUH $p < 0.001$; DEH $p < 0.001$), but the magnitude of change of thirst during the trial was different between conditions. Regarding fatigue, there was a trial effect ($F_{1,9} = 5.7$,

$p = 0.041$, $\eta^2 = 0.388$) and a time effect ($F_{1,9} = 21.8$, $p = 0.001$, $\eta^2 = 0.708$). The sensation of fatigue was higher at baseline of the DEH trial compared with EUH ($p = 0.016$), and fatigue increased over time in both trials (EUH $p = 0.050$; DEH $p = 0.003$). Analysis on concentration did not show any trial effect ($F_{1,9} = 1.6$, $p = 0.244$, $\eta^2 = 0.147$), but there was a time effect ($F_{1,9} = 32.7$, $p < 0.001$, $\eta^2 = 0.784$) and a time × trial effect ($F_{1,9} = 28.2$, $p < 0.001$, $\eta^2 = 0.758$). Concentration scores were lower at baseline of the DEH trial compared with the EUH trial ($p = 0.009$), but by the end of the trial, concentration feeling was similar between trials ($p = 0.320$) as this feeling was stable during the DEH trial ($p = 0.260$) and decreased in the EUH trial ($p < 0.001$). Analysis of alertness showed that there was no trial ($F_{1,9} = 1.7$, $p = 0.223$, $\eta^2 = 0.160$), no time effect ($F_{1,9} = 0.20$, $p = 0.660$, $\eta^2 = 0.023$), and neither a time × trial interaction ($F_{1,9} = 0.18$, $p = 0.678$, $\eta^2 = 0.020$).

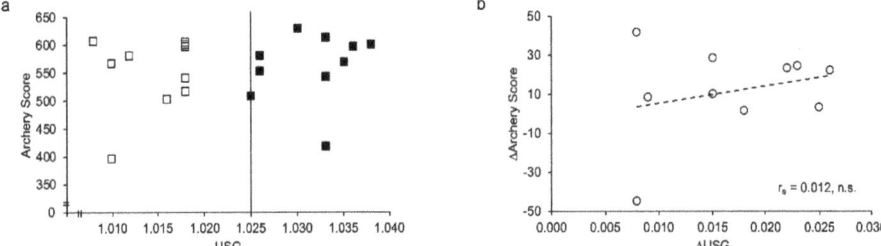

Figure 2. Archery Performance in relation to Urine Specific Gravity (USG) values. Panel (**a**) depicts both archery scores for EUH trial (open squares) and DEH trial (dark squares). Panel (**b**) depicts the correlation between ΔUSG ($USG_{DEH}-USG_{EUH}$) and ΔArchery score (Archery Score$_{DEH}$−Archery Score$_{EUH}$). No significant correlation was found between USG and Archery Performance.

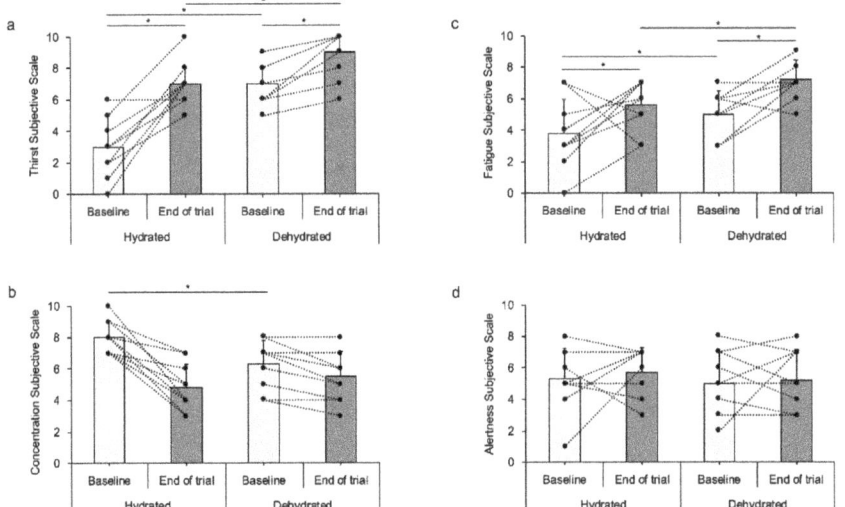

Figure 3. Subjective feelings of (**a**) Thirst, (**b**) Concentration, (**c**) Fatigue and (**d**) Alertness, at baseline and at the end of both Hydration (EUH) and Dehydration (DEH) trials. * Denotes statistically significant differences at the 0.05 level (2-tailed).

Heart rate response analysis (Figure 4) indicated a trial effect ($F_{1,9} = 9.9$, $p = 0.012$, $\eta^2 = 0.523$), and a time effect ($F_{13,117} = 136.3$, $p < 0.001$, $\eta^2 = 0.931$) as HR during the trial was above baseline in both conditions, and there was also a time × trial effect ($F_{13,117} = 2.2$, $p = 0.006$, $\eta^2 = 0.199$). Post hoc analysis showed that HR at baseline was higher in the DEH trial ($p = 0.003$), but it was similar during the first six throws ($p > 0.106$). During the short resting period after throw 6, HR remained elevated in the DEH trial compared with EUH trial ($p = 0.005$), and HR was significantly higher during the DEH trial at throws 7 ($p = 0.041$), 9 ($p = 0.043$), 10 ($p = 0.016$) and 11 ($p = 0.034$). The statistical difference between the two trials at throw 8 was $p = 0.086$ and at throw 12 $p = 0.075$, indicating a trend towards higher HR during the DEH trial.

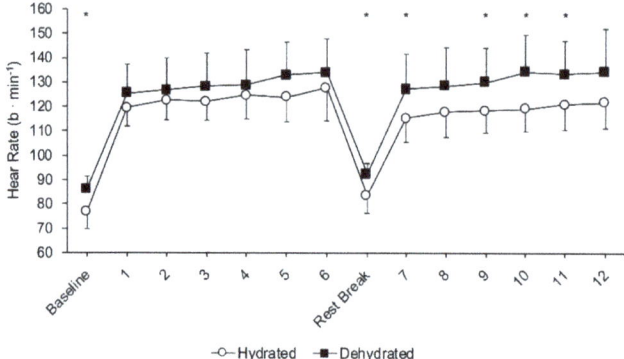

Figure 4. Heart rate response to hydration (open circles) and dehydration (dark squares) state, during the archery competition simulation. * Indicates difference between trials ($p < 0.050$). During exercise, heart rate was higher than baseline in both trials.

4. Discussion

In the current study, it was shown that dehydration induced psychological and physiological strain but did not alter shooting performance of national level archers during a competition simulation in hot environment. Specifically, the results of the current study indicate that archery score was not affected by dehydration. Nevertheless, significant differences on HR, subjective feelings of fatigue, and concentration were observed between conditions.

A compelling amount of evidence suggests that overall fitness, core strength, handgrip, upper body strength and static balance are related to archery performance and high scores [22,23]. In the present study, archery performance was similar between dehydration and euhydration trials; thereby, any potential effect on muscle function was not observed. Previous studies demonstrated that dehydration may decrease upper body muscle power during a maximum intensity anaerobic test [24] and during a fatiguing isometric strength protocol of repeated efforts at 85% of maximum voluntary contraction [7]. Nevertheless, the stress on the muscles during those tests was much higher than the effort during archery, and thus, it could be assumed that this is the reason why the participants in the present study were similarly successful during the two trials.

It has been proposed that the performance of experienced archers lies beyond their strength and fitness levels, to the mental domain, as the ability to concentrate is of utmost importance [25]. Dehydration may lead to impaired attention and motor coordination [26], decreased concentration [21,27,28] and increased sense of fatigue [21,28,29]. Additionally, dehydration has been linked to decreased sport-specific performance, such as decreased ball throwing accuracy in cricket [30] and basketball throw accuracy [31]. Mental fatigue has been shown to impair tennis serve and ground strokes accuracy [32]. The effects of dehydration may be more intense in hot and humid conditions due to a potentially increased thermal strain, which can affect the nervous system, cerebral blood flow and increase mental fatigue [33]. In this investigation, participants reported that they felt less able to concentrate and more fatigued at the dehydration baseline. Despite these relatively negative feelings, the overall archery score was not affected, even though the trials took place under conditions of high ambient temperature and humidity. Literature shows that experienced archers have higher emotional intelligence and emotional regulation;

thereby, under stressful conditions, they may respond with higher consistency in cognitive processes during shooting [34].

Except for the induced psychological burden, dehydration had a significant physiological effect on the participants cardiovascular system. During the dehydration trial, heart rate was higher at baseline and during the second half of the competition simulation. In response to dehydration, heart rate may rise in order to maintain blood pressure and oxygen delivery [35]. A higher heart rate has been shown to increase tremors [36], which can potentially affect shooting performance. Indeed, higher heart rate has been associated with decreased performance in pistol shooting [37] and archery performance [14,38], since target aiming requires great stability by the archers and a high level of hand-eye coordination. Although archery performance was not affected over 72 arrow throws in the present study, during an official competition this volume of arrow throws equates to half of the anticipated number of throws until a winner is decided. Thus, as heart rate increased significantly during the latter stages of this investigation, it is unknown whether the magnitude of these changes in heart rate and aiming precision would be greater during a longer official competition with 140 arrow throws. Therefore, archers are advised to follow the current recommendations for fluid intake during exercise according to ACSM guidelines [39].

To the best of our knowledge, no study to date explored the effect of dehydration on archery performance in the field. Although it falls beyond the scope of the present study, it could be interesting to investigate the mediating effect of hormonal responses during this dehydration scenario into a larger sample size. Furthermore, as self-perceived psychological burden may compromise performance, a long-term observational investigation of hydration status and performance in archers would be of great value and could possibly elucidate physiological adaptations, underlying the current results. In addition, future studies on archery could include examination of secondary variables such as grip strength, or cognitive tests, in order to gain knowledge on specific physiological mechanisms or sports performance related parameters which can be affected by dehydration.

Limitations of the study. Potential limitations of the present study include the small sample size and absence of blood dehydration markers or body mass changes during the trials. Although urine specific gravity might not be the gold standard, the values of USG > 1.030 recorded in the present study, following fluid restriction, are a clear indication that dehydration was above 2% body mass [20], the critical dehydration point for athletic performance. Additionally, fluid restriction cannot be blunted in a real-world scenario. However, the strength of the present study lies on the fact that this is probably the first study in literature to directly address potential dehydration effects on advanced archers in a simulated competition, following controlled dehydration via fluid restriction.

5. Conclusions

To conclude, dehydration induced psychological and physiological strain in national level archers, revealed by decreased feeling of concentration, increased sensation of fatigue and increased heart rate during a competition simulation in a hot environment. The degree of this added burden did not affect archery performance over 72 arrow throws. Further investigation is required to elucidate the effect of the observed increased heart rate over time during the dehydration trial, which could potentially have a negative impact on aiming precision and archery performance over a complete competition with 140 arrow throws.

Author Contributions: Conceptualization, G.A., A.S. and C.D.G.; investigation, A.S., P.S.S. and A.V.; resources, G.A.; data curation, G.A. and C.D.G.; writing—original draft preparation, G.A. and A.S.; writing—review and editing, G.A., C.D.G., A.V. and P.S.S.; supervision, G.A. All authors have read and agreed to the published version of the manuscript.

Funding: This research received no external funding.

Conflicts of Interest: The authors declare no conflict of interest.

References

1. Cheuvront, S.N.; Kenefick, R.W. Dehydration: Physiology, Assessment, and Performance Effects. *Compr. Physiol.* **2014**, *4*, 257–285. [CrossRef] [PubMed]
2. Cheuvront, S.N.; Carter, R.; Sawka, M.N. Fluid Balance and Endurance Exercise Performance. *Curr. Sports Med. Rep.* **2003**, *2*, 202–208. [CrossRef] [PubMed]
3. Green, J.M.; Miller, B.; Simpson, J.; Dubroc, D.; Keyes, A.; Neal, K.; Gann, J.; Andre, T. Effects of 2% Dehydration on Lactate Concentration During Constant-Load Cycling. *J. Strength Cond. Res. Natl. Strength Cond. Assoc.* **2018**, *32*, 2066–2071. [CrossRef] [PubMed]
4. Armstrong, L.E.; Costill, D.L.; Fink, W.J. Influence of diuretic-induced dehydration on competitive running performance. *Med. Sci. Sports Exerc.* **1985**, *17*, 456–461. [CrossRef] [PubMed]
5. Slater, G.J.; Rice, A.J.; Tanner, R.; Sharpe, K.; Jenkins, D.G.; Hahn, A.G. Impact of Two Different Body Mass Management Strategies on Repeat Rowing Performance. *Med. Sci. Sports Exerc.* **2006**, *38*, 138–146. [CrossRef] [PubMed]
6. Nuccio, R.P.; Barnes, K.A.; Carter, J.M.; Baker, L.B. Fluid Balance in Team Sport Athletes and the Effect of Hypohydration on Cognitive, Technical, and Physical Performance. *Sports Med. (Auckl. N. Z.)* **2017**, *47*, 1951–1982. [CrossRef] [PubMed]
7. Barley, O.; Chapman, D.W.; Blazevich, A.J.; Abbiss, C.R. Acute Dehydration Impairs Endurance without Modulating Neuromuscular Function. *Front. Physiol.* **2018**, *9*, 9. [CrossRef]
8. Judelson, D.A.; Maresh, C.M.; Farrell, M.J.; Yamamoto, L.M.; Armstrong, L.E.; Kraemer, W.J.; Volek, J.S.; Spiering, B.A.; Casa, D.J.; Anderson, J.M. Effect of Hydration State on Strength, Power, and Resistance Exercise Performance. *Med. Sci. Sports Exerc.* **2007**, *39*, 1817–1824. [CrossRef]
9. Lin, J.-J.; Hung, C.-J.; Yang, C.-C.; Chen, H.-Y.; Chou, F.-C.; Lu, T.-W. Activation and tremor of the shoulder muscles to the demands of an archery task. *J. Sports Sci.* **2010**, *28*, 415–421. [CrossRef]
10. Shinohara, H.; Urabe, Y. Analysis of muscular activity in archery: A comparison of skill level. *J. Sports Med. Phys. Fit.* **2018**, *58*, 1752–1758. [CrossRef]
11. Nishizono, H.; Nakagawa, K.; Suda, T.; Saito, K. An electromyographical analysis of purposive muscle activity and appearance of muscle silent period in archery shooting. *Jpn. J. Phys. Fit. Sports Med.* **1984**, *33*, 17–26. [CrossRef]
12. Gauchard, G.C.; Gangloff, P.; Vouriot, A.; Mallié, J.-P.; Perrin, P.P. Effects of exercise-induced fatigue with and without hydration on static postural control in adult human subjects. *Int. J. Neurosci.* **2002**, *112*, 1191–1206. [CrossRef] [PubMed]
13. Carrillo, A.E.; Christodoulou, V.X.; Koutedakis, Y.; Flouris, A.D. Autonomic nervous system modulation during an archery competition in novice and experienced adolescent archers. *J. Sports Sci.* **2011**, *29*, 913–917. [CrossRef] [PubMed]
14. Robazza, C.; Bortoli, L.; Nougier, V. Emotions, heart rate and performance in archery. A case study. *J. sports Med. Phys. Fit.* **1999**, *39*, 169–176.
15. Helin, P.; Sihvonen, T.; Hänninen, O. Timing of the triggering action of shooting in relation to the cardiac cycle. *Br. J. Sports Med.* **1987**, *21*, 33–36. [CrossRef]
16. Dieleman, N.; Koek, H.L.; Hendrikse, J. Short-term mechanisms influencing volumetric brain dynamics. *NeuroImage Clin.* **2017**, *16*, 507–513. [CrossRef]
17. Kempton, M.J.; Ettinger, U.; Foster, R.; Williams, S.; Calvert, G.A.; Hampshire, A.; Zelaya, F.; O'Gorman, R.; McMorris, T.; Owen, A.M.; et al. Dehydration affects brain structure and function in healthy adolescents. *Hum. Brain Mapp.* **2010**, *32*, 71–79. [CrossRef]
18. Ganio, M.S.; Armstrong, L.E.; Casa, U.J.; McDermott, B.P.; Lee, E.C.; Yamamoto, L.M.; Marzano, S.; Lopez, R.M.; Jimenez, L.; Le Bellego, L.; et al. Mild dehydration impairs cognitive performance and mood of men. *Br. J. Nutr.* **2011**, *106*, 1535–1543. [CrossRef]
19. D'Anci, K.E.; Mahoney, C.R.; Vibhakar, A.; Kanter, J.H.; Taylor, H.A. Voluntary Dehydration and Cognitive Performance in Trained College Athletes. *Percept. Mot. Ski.* **2009**, *109*, 251–269. [CrossRef]
20. Cheuvront, S.N.; Ely, B.R.; Kenefick, R.W.; Sawka, M.N. Biological variation and diagnostic accuracy of dehydration assessment markers. *Am. J. Clin. Nutr.* **2010**, *92*, 565–573. [CrossRef]
21. Shirreffs, S.M.; Merson, S.J.; Fraser, S.M.; Archer, D.T. The effects of fluid restriction on hydration status and subjective feelings in man. *Br. J. Nutr.* **2004**, *91*, 951–958. [CrossRef] [PubMed]

22. Martin, P.E.; Siler, W.L.; Hoffman, D. Electromyographic analysis of bow string release in highly skilled archers. *J. Sports Sci.* **1990**, *8*, 215–221. [CrossRef] [PubMed]
23. Ertan, H.; Kentel, B.B.; Tümer, S.T.; Korkusuz, F. Activation patterns in forearm muscles during archery shooting. *Hum. Mov. Sci.* **2003**, *22*, 37–45. [CrossRef]
24. Jones, L.C.; Cleary, M.A.; Lopez, R.M.; Zuri, R.E.; Lopez, R. Active Dehydration Impairs Upper and Lower Body Anaerobic Muscular Power. *J. Strength Cond. Res.* **2008**, *22*, 455–463. [CrossRef] [PubMed]
25. Kim, H.-B.; Kim, S.-H.; So, W.-Y. The Relative Importance of Performance Factors in Korean Archery. *J. Strength Cond. Res.* **2015**, *29*, 1211–1219. [CrossRef] [PubMed]
26. Wittbrodt, M.; Millard-Stafford, M. Dehydration Impairs Cognitive Performance: A Meta-analysis. *Med. Sci. Sports Exerc.* **2018**, *50*, 2360–2368. [CrossRef] [PubMed]
27. Szinnai, G.; Schachinger, H.; Arnaud, M.J.; Linder, L.; Keller, U. Effect of water deprivation on cognitive-motor performance in healthy men and women. *Am. J. Physiol. Integr. Comp. Physiol.* **2005**, *289*, R275–R280. [CrossRef]
28. Stavrinou, P.S.; Giannaki, C.D.; Andreou, E.; Aphamis, G. Prevalence of hypohydration in adolescents during the school day in Cyprus: Seasonal variations. *East. Mediterr. Health J.* **2020**, *26*. [CrossRef]
29. Aphamis, G.; Stavrinou, P.; Andreou, E.; Giannaki, C.D. Hydration status, total water intake and subjective feelings of adolescents living in a hot environment, during a typical school day. *Int. J. Adolesc. Med. Health* **2019**. [CrossRef]
30. Gamage, J.P.; De Silva, A.P.; Nalliah, A.K.; Galloway, S.D. Effects of Dehydration on Cricket Specific Skill Performance in Hot and Humid Conditions. *Int. J. Sport Nutr. Exerc. Metab.* **2016**, *26*, 531–541. [CrossRef]
31. Baker, L.B.; Dougherty, K.A.; Chow, M.; Kenney, W.L. Progressive Dehydration Causes a Progressive Decline in Basketball Skill Performance. *Med. Sci. Sports Exerc.* **2007**, *39*, 1114–1123. [CrossRef] [PubMed]
32. Le Mansec, Y.; Pageaux, B.; Nordez, A.; Dorel, S.; Jubeau, M. Mental fatigue alters the speed and the accuracy of the ball in table tennis. *J. Sports Sci.* **2017**, *36*, 1–9. [CrossRef] [PubMed]
33. Nybo, L.; Rasmussen, P.; Sawka, M.N. Performance in the Heat-Physiological Factors of Importance for Hyperthermia-Induced Fatigue. *Compr. Physiol.* **2014**, *4*, 657–689. [CrossRef] [PubMed]
34. Chang, Y.; Lee, J.-J.; Seo, J.-H.; Song, H.-J.; Kim, Y.-T.; Lee, H.J.; Kim, H.J.; Lee, J.; Kim, W.; Woo, M.; et al. Neural correlates of motor imagery for elite archers. *NMR Biomed.* **2010**, *24*, 366–372. [CrossRef] [PubMed]
35. Castro-Sepulveda, M.; Cerda-Kohler, H.; Pérez-Luco, C.; Monsalves-Alvarez, M.; Andrade, D.C.; Zbinden-Foncea, H.; Martín, E.B.-S.; Ramírez-Campillo, R. Hydration status after exercise affect resting metabolic rate and heart rate variability. *Nutr. Hosp.* **2014**, *31*, 1273–1277.
36. Lakie, M. The influence of muscle tremor on shooting performance. *Exp. Physiol.* **2010**, *95*, 441–450. [CrossRef]
37. Fenici, R.; Ruggieri, M.P.; Brisinda, D.; Fenici, P. Cardiovascular adaptation during action pistol shooting. *J. Sports Med. Phys. Fit.* **1999**, *39*, 259–266.
38. Clemente, F.; Couceiro, M.; Rocha, R.; Mendes, R. Study of the Heart Rate and Accuracy Performance of Archers. *J. Phys. Educ. Sport* **2011**, *11*, 434–437.
39. Sawka, M.N.; Burke, L.M.; Eichner, E.R.; Maughan, R.J.; Montain, S.J.; Stachenfeld, N.S. American College of Sports Medicine position stand. Exercise and fluid replacement. *Med. Sci. Sports Exerc.* **2007**, *39*, 377–390. [CrossRef]

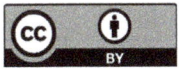

© 2020 by the authors. Licensee MDPI, Basel, Switzerland. This article is an open access article distributed under the terms and conditions of the Creative Commons Attribution (CC BY) license (http://creativecommons.org/licenses/by/4.0/).

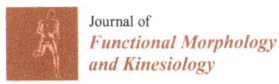

Brief Report

Bioimpedance Vector References Need to Be Period-Specific for Assessing Body Composition and Cellular Health in Elite Soccer Players: A Brief Report

Tindaro Bongiovanni [1,2], Gabriele Mascherini [3,*], Federico Genovesi [4], Giulio Pasta [5], Fedon Marcello Iaia [2], Athos Trecroci [2], Marco Ventimiglia [6], Giampietro Alberti [2] and Francesco Campa [7]

1. Department of Health, Performance and Recovery, Parma Calcio 1913, 40121 Parma, Italy; tindaro.bongiovanni@gmail.com
2. Department of Biomedical Sciences for Health, Università degli Studi di Milano, 20129 Milano, Italy; marcello.iaia@unimi.it (F.M.I.); Athos.Trecroci@unimi.it (A.T.); gianpietro.alberti@unimi.it (G.A.)
3. Department of Experimental and Clinical Medicine, Università degli Studi di Firenze, 50139 Florence, Italy
4. Medical Department Manchester City Football Club, Manchester 03101, UK; fede.genovesi@libero.it
5. Medical Department Parma Calcio 1913, 40121 Parma, Italy; ghitopasta@hotmail.com
6. Inflammatory Bowel Disease Unit, A.O.O.R. Villa Sofia-Cervello, 90146 Palermo, Italy; marco.ventimiglia@unipa.it
7. Department for Life Quality Studies, University of Bologna, 47921 Rimini, Italy; francesco.campa3@unibo.it
* Correspondence: gabriele.mascherini@unifi.it

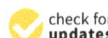

Received: 27 August 2020; Accepted: 29 September 2020; Published: 1 October 2020

Abstract: Purpose: Bioimpedance data through bioimpedance vector analysis (BIVA) is used to evaluate cellular function and body fluid content. This study aimed to (i) identify whether BIVA patters differ according to the competitive period and (ii) provide specific references for assessing bioelectric properties at the start of the season in male elite soccer players. Methods: The study included 131 male soccer players (age: 25.1 ± 4.7 yr, height: 183.4 ± 6.1 cm, weight: 79.3 ± 6.6) registered in the first Italian soccer division (Serie A). Bioimpedance analysis was performed just before the start of the competitive season and BIVA was applied. In order to verify the need for period-specific references, bioelectrical values measured at the start of the season were compared to the reference values for the male elite soccer player population. Results: The results of the two-sample Hotelling T^2 tests showed that in the bivariate interpretation of the raw bioimpedance parameters (resistance (R) and reactance (Xc)) the bioelectric properties significantly ($T^2 = 15.3$, $F = 7.6$, $p \leq 0.001$, Mahalanobis D = 0.45) differ between the two phases of the competition analyzed. In particular, the mean impedance vector is more displaced to the left into the R-Xc graph at the beginning of the season than in the first half of the championship. Conclusions: For an accurate evaluation of body composition and cellular health, the tolerance ellipses displayed by BIVA approach into the R-Xc graph must be period-specific. This study provides new specific tolerance ellipses (R/H: 246 ± 32.1, Xc/H: 34.3 ± 5.1, r: 0.7) for performing BIVA at the beginning of the competitive season in male elite soccer players.

Keywords: BIVA; phase angle; R-Xc graph; tolerance ellipses

1. Introduction

Body composition analysis is currently one of the most studied evaluations in sport, mainly for the relationship between physical characteristics and sports performance [1]. In sports, excess fat mass reduces endurance performance, while an increase in lean mass, especially muscle mass, is associated with an increase in power and strength [2]. Furthermore, the assessment of localized body composition allows the identification of differences in muscle mass and strength between areas of the body and may allow a reduction in the risk of injury (evaluation of contralateral limbs, agonist-antagonists) [3].

Body composition assessment should also be considered in sports involving weight categories, where athletes benefit from being placed in a lower weight category, in these cases any weight loss must therefore be monitored closely. Excessive training coupled with calorie restrictions can lead to excessive, unnecessary and dangerous weight loss. This weight loss in both women and men decreases performance, bone mineral density, muscle mass and is detrimental to health [4,5].

Bioelectrical impedance vector analysis (BIVA) is a method widely used to evaluate body composition and cellular health in athletes, as well as in the general population [6–9]. This method considers the raw bioelectrical parameters (resistance and reactance) standardized for the height of the subjects as a vector within a graph. Resistance (R) is the opposition to the flow of an injected alternating current, at any current frequency, through intra- and extra-cellular ionic solutions, while reactance (Xc) represents the dielectric or capacitive component of cell membranes and organelles, and tissue interfaces [10].

BIVA allows for the monitoring of vector changes over time or the comparison of the vector position within the R-Xc graph on specific population tolerance ellipses [11–13]. Given the ease and repeatability of this method, several references for athletes have recently been proposed, including those for soccer players [14], volleyball players [15], and cyclists [16], while also considering the competitive level of the athlete.

In soccer, Levi Micheli et al. [14] were the first to demonstrate how athletes need to be assessed on specific tolerance ellipses, showing bioelectric values that were far different than those of the normal healthy population. Subsequently, Mascherini et al. [17] suggested how bioimpedance vectors show displacements over the season, reflecting the changes that occur in the body composition and physical condition of the players. This was later confirmed by Campa et al. [18] who analyzed the bioelectrical changes comparing BIVA to results obtained by Dual X-ray Absorptiometry (DXA) and dilution techniques over a season in athletes, also showing that these vector changes occur in many other sports.

During the different phases of competition, the one which precedes the start of the season is among the most important periods in which to evaluate the athlete's physical condition and the body composition adjustments that are sought during the pre-season. Considering the vector changes that occur over the season, the bioelectrical references used in the BIVA assessment must be specific for the competitive period in which the athlete is tested. Therefore, the purpose of this study was to show how BIVA references provided in different phases of the season differ in male elite soccer players, also providing new references for assessing body composition in the start-of-the season period.

2. Materials and Methods

2.1. Design and Participants

A total of 131 male professional soccer players (age: 25.1 ± 4.7 yr; height: 183.4 ± 6.1 cm; weight: 79.3 ± 6.6 Kg) were recruited and participated in this observational study.

The inclusion criteria were: (1) players registered and participating in the first (Serie A) Italian National division; (2) non-injured at the time of the assessment. After having been informed about the aims and the procedures of the research, all athletes gave their written informed consent. The project was approved by the Bioethics Committee of the University of Milan (approval code: 1052019) and was conducted in accordance with the guidelines of the declaration of Helsinki.

2.2. Procedures

All measurements were performed in resting and fasting conditions at the facilities of the teams in the last week of August at 8.30 a.m. Generally, this period corresponds to the end of the preparation for the competitive season; therefore, it coincides with the start of the season. Body height was recorded to the nearest 0.1 cm with a stadiometer (SECA® 240, Hamburg, Germany) and weight was measured to the nearest 0.1 Kg with a calibrated weight scales (SECA® 877, Hamburg, Germany).

Whole-body impedance was obtained using a bioimpedance analyzer (BIA 101 Anniversary Edition, Akern, Florence, Italy). The device emits an alternating sinusoidal electric current of 400 mA at an operating single frequency of 50 kHz (±0.1%). Subjects were positioned with a leg opening of 45° with respect to the midline of the body, and with the upper limbs positioned 30° away from the trunk. The bioelectric phase angle (PhA) was calculated as the arctangent of Xc/R × 180/π. BIVA was carried out using the classic methods, e.g., normalizing R (ohm) and Xc (ohm) for height in meters [6,8].

2.3. Statistical Analyses

The two-sample Hotelling T^2 test was used to compare the differences in the mean impedance vectors between the bioimpedance data measured on the athletes of this study and the reference bioelectric values proposed by Levi Micheli et al. [14] The 50, 75, and 95% tolerance ellipses were generated using the BIVA software [19]. Statistical significance was predetermined as $p < 0.05$. Data were analyzed with IBM SPSS Statistics, version 24.0 (IBM Corp., Armonk, NY, USA).

3. Results

Table 1 shows anthropometric and bioelectrical characteristics of the soccer player.

Table 1. Descriptive statistics for the soccer players according to playing position.

Variable	Goalkeepers n = (15)	Defenders n = (38)	Midfielders n = (38)	Forwards n = (40)	All n = (131)
Age (years)	24.2 ± 5.9	26.6 ± 4.8	25.0 ± 4.8	24.5 ± 3.9	25.1 ± 4.7
Weight (kg)	86.7 ± 5.4	80.6 ± 5.6	76.8 ± 5.6	77.6 ± 6.5	79.3 ± 6.6
Height (cm)	188.3 ± 3.5	185.1 ± 5.0	181.4 ± 5.2	181.8 ± 7.2	181.8 ± 7.2
BMI (kg/m^2)	24.5 ± 1.0	23.5 ± 0.8	23.3 ± 1.0	23.5 ± 1.0	23.5 ± 1.0
R/H (ohm/m)	234.0 ± 18.1	242.9 ± 17.0	251.9 ± 18.9	254.6 ± 21.9	248.1 ± 20.3
Xc/H (ohm/m)	33.0 ± 3.9	34.4 ± 3.1	34.7 ± 3.2	35.4 ± 3.0	34.6 ± 3.3
PhA (degree)	8.0 ± 0.7	8.1 ± 0.5	7.8 ± 0.4	7.9 ± 0.4	8.0 ± 0.5

Abbreviations: BMI, body mass index; R/H, resistance standardized for height; Xc/H, reactance standardized for height; PhA, phase angle.

The results of the two-sample Hotelling's T^2 test showed separate 95% confidence ellipses indicating a significant difference ($T^2 = 15.3$, F = 7.6, $p \leq 0.001$, Mahalanobis D = 0.45) between the BIVA patters measured in this study and those proposed by Levi Micheli et al. [14] as a reference for the male elite soccer players population (Figure 1a).

The new reference ellipses and the single bioimpedance vectors measured in the soccer players at the start of the season are shown in Figure 1b.

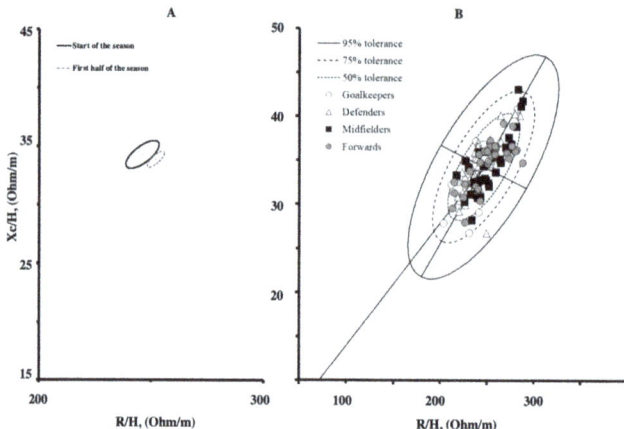

Figure 1. Mean impedance vectors with the 95% confidence ellipses for the soccer players measured at the start and at the first half of the competitive season [10] (Panel **A**). Scattergrams of the individual impedance vectors plotted on the new tolerance ellipses (Panel **B**).

4. Discussion

The aim of this study was to show the importance of evaluating bioelectric properties using BIVA references that are suitable for the competitive period in which the assessment is carried out. The results of this study, which provide bioelectrical impedance data for 131 elite players, showed how the tolerance ellipses created on the basis of measurements during the different phases of the competition differ significantly for elite soccer players.

The bioimpedance data reported in the present study are comparable to previous values reported during the start-of-the season period in elite soccer players [20–22]. In comparison with the elite Italian male soccer population investigated by Levi Micheli et al. [14], the elite soccer players measured in this study showed a significant vector shift to the left on the minor axis of the tolerance ellipses. This could indicate a greater cell mass, which is a consequence of the effects sought in the preparation phase (training and controlled diet) typically, designed to increase endurance level and increase strength [23]. In fact, in a previous study, Mascherini et al. [17] suggested that the shortening of the vector was associated with changes in hydration status and increases in body cell mass. In this study, the preparation phase could have increased the intracellular/extracellular water (ICW/ECW) ratio as can be seen from a higher PhA than that measured by Levi Micheli et al. [14] (8.0 ± 0.5° vs. 7.7 ± 0.6°). Indeed, PhA is positively associated with the ICW/ECW ratio in athletes [18,24]. Bioelectric data reflect the content of body fluids and the cellular health of the athlete and during the season, which change in response to training load and physical condition over the season [25]. In fact, the new tolerance ellipses proposed in this study differ significantly from those generated in the study by Levi Micheli et al. [14], in which bioimpedance measurements were collected in the first half of the competitive period. Furthermore, Micheli Levi et al. [14] reported that BIA data was collected over 5 months, from October to January 2009–2010, a period of time that may have generated vector changes in the athletes themselves. Our hypothesis is that the increase in workload (training) and official matches from August to October (about 6–8 matches played) or from August to January (16–17 matches played) could lead to fatigue and increased muscle turnover, as well as reduced muscle function which could result in a shift to the right of the biompedance vector. In fact, during the season, the reduction of the PhA could indicate a decreased muscle function as shown by Norman et al. [26] However, since we have not performed any muscle function tests, this hypothesis will have to be further investigated in future studies.

The reference ellipses proposed in the literature for athletes are population-specific. In addition to those for soccer players proposed by Levi Micheli [14], Campa and Toselli [15] measured male volleyball players in the second half of the in-season and showed specific BIA vector distribution in elite players in comparison to lower levels athletes. Subsequently, Giorgi et al. [16] provided bioelectrical impedance data of male road cyclists of varying performance levels, measured at the time of their optimal performance level and identified the 50, 75 and 95% tolerance ellipses for the road cyclists population, as well as for the high-performance road cyclists. In addition to these, there are also ellipses for healthy athletes built on more than 1000 male and 440 female athletes during the off-season period, therefore suitable for evaluating BIVA in the first phase of the competitive season [12].

The authors are also aware of the limitations of the study. Firstly, the subjects come from the same territory; therefore, the results obtained are not generalizable to all the soccer players around the world: a larger sample size is required even in different countries. The second is that no division by ethnicity of the players has been made in order to obtain a sample as large as possible: currently an international data collection is active that will allow us to investigate both these two limitations.

A strength of this study is in the specific time period in which the measurements were collected, not only in regard to the competitive level of the athletes, but above all for the time span in which BIA assessments were performed. In fact, BIA measurements were collected within a week, just before the start of the season, a period of time too short to generate vector changes between the players.

For the reasons mentioned above, future studies conducted with the aim of providing BIVA references for athletes should carry out the measurements according to the competitive phase for which they want to provide the new references. This is very significative given that vector changes occur during the different phases of the season in athletes, and bioelectrical values must be as informative and specific as possible, in order to obtain accurate monitoring of the body composition and physical condition of the athlete. This study demonstrates the importance of evaluating athletes on period-specific BIVA references, providing new tolerance ellipses for assessing body composition and cellular health before the start of the competitive season in elite soccer players.

5. Conclusions

Through BIVA, it is possible to evaluate body composition and the state of physical condition in the different phases of the competition in elite soccer players. This study provides specific BIVA references for the start of the season period, through which the physical condition achieved after the preparation micro cycle in soccer can be assessed.

Author Contributions: Conceptualization, F.C. and G.M.; methodology, T.B.; software, F.C.; validation, F.M.I., G.P.; formal analysis, F.C.; investigation, T.B.; data curation, F.G.; writing—original draft preparation, F.C. and G.M.; supervision, A.T. and M.V.; project administration, G.A. All authors have read and agreed to the published version of the manuscript.

Funding: This research received no external funding.

Acknowledgments: The authors are grateful to all the soccer players who took part in this study.

Conflicts of Interest: The authors declare no conflict of interest.

References

1. Bongiovanni, T.; Trecroci, A.; Cavaggioni, L.; Rossi, A.; Perri, E.; Pasta, G.; Iaia, F.M.; Alberti, G. Importance of anthropometric features to predict physical performance in elite youth soccer: A machine learning approach. *Res. Sports Med.* **2020**, 1–12. [CrossRef] [PubMed]
2. Campa, F.; Semprini, G.; Júdice, P.B.; Messina, G.; Toselli, S. Anthropometry, Physical and Movement Features, and Repeated-sprint Ability in Soccer Players. *Int. J. Sports Med.* **2019**, *40*, 100–109. [CrossRef] [PubMed]
3. Ackland, T.R.; Lohman, T.G.; Sundgot-Borgen, J.; Maughan, R.J.; Meyer, N.L.; Stewart, A.D.; Müller, W. Current status of body composition assessment in sport: Review and position statement on behalf of the ad hoc research working group on body composition health and performance, under the auspices of the I.O.C. Medical Commission. *Sports Med.* **2012**, *42*, 227–249. [CrossRef] [PubMed]

4. Nattiv, A.; Loucks, A.B.; Manore, M.M.; Sanborn, C.F.; Sundgot-Borgen, J.; Warren, M.P.; American College of Sports Medicine. American College of Sports Medicine position stand. The female athlete triad. *Med. Sci. Sports Exerc.* **2007**, *39*, 1867–1882. [CrossRef]
5. Galanti, G.; Bocci, M.; Petri, C.; Tempesti, G.; Mascherini, G. Body composition analysis as a health index in cyclists. *Med. Dello Sport* **2018**, *71*, 75–85. [CrossRef]
6. Mascherini, G.; Cattozzo, A.; Petri, C.; Francini, L.; Galanti, G. Application of Bioelectrical Vector Analysis in Professional Soccer Players: BIVA in sport. In Proceedings of the 2nd International Congress on Sports Sciences Research and Technology Support (icSPORTS-2014), Rome, Italy, 24–26 October 2014; Science and Technology Publications: Setúbal, Portugal; pp. 84–88. [CrossRef]
7. Castizo-Olier, J.; Irurtia, A.; Jemni, M.; Carrasco-Marginet, M.; Fernández-García, R.; Rodríguez, F.A. Bioelectrical impedance vector analysis (BIVA) in sport and exercise: Systematic review and future perspectives. *PLoS ONE* **2018**, *13*, e0197957. [CrossRef]
8. dos Santos, L.; Ribeiro, A.S.; Gobbo, L.A.; Nunes, J.P.; Cunha, P.M.; Campa, F.; Toselli, S.; Schoenfeld, B.J.; Sardinha, L.B.; Cyrino, E.S. Effects of Resistance Training with Different Pyramid Systems on Bioimpedance Vector Patterns, Body Composition, and Cellular Health in Older Women: A Randomized Controlled Trial. *Sustainability* **2020**, *12*, 6658. [CrossRef]
9. Toselli, S.; Badicu, G.; Bragonzoni, L.; Spiga, F.; Mazzuca, P.; Campa, F. Comparison of the effect of different resistance training frequencies on phase angle and handgrip strength in obese women: A randomized controlled trial. *Int. J. Environ. Res. Public Health* **2020**, *17*, 1163. [CrossRef]
10. Lukaski, H.C.; Piccoli, A. Bioelectrical Impedance Vector Analysis for Assessment of Hydration in Physiological States and Clinical Conditions. In *Handbook of Anthropometry*; Preedy, V., Ed.; Springer: Berlin/Heidelberg, Germany, 2012; pp. 287–305.
11. Campa, F.; Gatterer, H.; Lukaski, H.; Toselli, S. Stabilizing bioimpedance-vector-analysis measures with a 10-min cold shower after running exercise to enable assessment of body hydration. *Int. J. Sports Physiol. Perform.* **2019**, *14*, 1006–1009. [CrossRef]
12. Campa, F.; Matias, C.; Gatterer, H.; Toselli, S.; Koury, J.C.; Andreoli, A.; Melchiorri, G.; Sardinha, L.B.; Silva, A.M. Classic bioelectrical impedance vector reference values for assessing body composition in male and female athletes. *Int. J. Environ. Res. Public Health* **2019**, *16*, 5066. [CrossRef]
13. Koury, J.C.; Trugo, M.F.N.; Torres, A.G. Phase angle and bioelectrical impedance vectors in adolescent and adult male athletes. *Int. J. Sports Physiol. Perform.* **2014**, *9*, 798–804. [CrossRef] [PubMed]
14. Levi Micheli, M.; Pagani, L.; Marella, M.; Gulisano, M.; Piccoli, A.; Angelini, F.; Burtscher, M.; Gatterer, H. Bioimpedance and impedance vector patterns as predictors of league level in male soccer players. *Int. J. Sports Physiol. Perform.* **2014**, *9*, 532–539. [CrossRef] [PubMed]
15. Campa, F.; Toselli, S. Bioimpedance vector analysis of elite, subelite, and low-level male volleyball players. *Int. J. Sports Physiol. Perform.* **2018**, *13*, 1250–1253. [CrossRef]
16. Giorgi, A.; Vicini, M.; Pollastri, L.; Lombardi, E.; Magni, E.; Andreazzoli, A.; Orsini, M.; Bonifazi, M.; Lukaski, H.; Gatterer, H. Bioimpedance patterns and bioelectrical impedance vector analysis (BIVA) of road cyclists. *J. Sports Sci.* **2018**, *36*, 2608–2613. [CrossRef] [PubMed]
17. Mascherini, G.; Gatterer, H.; Lukaski, H.; Burtscher, M.; Galanti, G. Changes in hydration, body-cell mass and endurance performance of professional soccer players through a competitive season. *J. Sports Med. Phys. Fit.* **2015**, *55*, 749–755.
18. Campa, F.; Matias, C.N.; Marini, E.; Heymsfield, S.B.; Toselli, S.; Sardinha, L.B.; Silva, A.M. Identifying athlete body-fluid changes during a competitive season with bioelectrical impedance vector analysis. *Int. J. Sports Physiol. Perform.* **2020**, *15*, 361–367. [CrossRef]
19. Piccoli, A.; Pastori, G. *BIVA Software*; Department of Medical and Surgical Sciences, University of Padova: Padova, Italy, 2002.
20. Mascherini, G.; Castizo-Olier, J.; Irurtia, A.; Petri, C.; Galanti, G. Differences between the sexes in athletes' body composition and lower limb bioimpedance values. *Muscles Ligaments Tendons J.* **2018**, *7*, 573–581.
21. Mascherini, G.; Petri, C.; Galanti, G. Integrated total body composition and localized fat-free mass assessment. *Sport Sci. Health* **2015**, *11*, 217–225. [CrossRef]
22. Petri, C.; Mascherini, G.; Bini, V.; Anania, G.; Calà, P.; Toncelli, L.; Galanti, G. Integrated total body composition versus Body Mass Index in young athletes. *Minerva Pediatr.* **2020**, *72*, 163–169. [CrossRef]

23. Gregson, W.; Littlewood, M. Science in Soccer. In *Translating Theory into Practice*; Bloomsburry Publishing Plc: London, UK, 2018.
24. Marini, E.; Campa, F.; Buffa, R.; Stagi, S.; Matias, C.N.; Toselli, S.; Sardinha, L.B.; Silva, A.M. Phase angle and bioelectrical impedance vector analysis in the evaluation of body composition in athletes. *Clin. Nutr.* **2020**, *39*, 447–454. [CrossRef]
25. Reis, J.F.; Matias, C.N.; Campa, F.; Morgado, J.P.; Franco, P.; Quaresma, P.; Almeida, N.; Curto, D.; Toselli, S.; Monteiro, C.P. Bioimpedance Vector Patterns Changes in Response to Swimming Training: An Ecological Approach. *Int. J. Environ. Res. Public Health* **2020**, *17*, 4851. [CrossRef] [PubMed]
26. Norman, K.; Stobäus, N.; Pirlich, M.; Bosy-Westphal, A. Bioelectrical phase angle and impedance vector analysis—Clinical relevance and applicability of impedance parameters. *Clin. Nutr.* **2012**, *31*, 854–861. [CrossRef] [PubMed]

Publisher's Note: MDPI stays neutral with regard to jurisdictional claims in published maps and institutional affiliations.

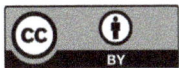

© 2020 by the authors. Licensee MDPI, Basel, Switzerland. This article is an open access article distributed under the terms and conditions of the Creative Commons Attribution (CC BY) license (http://creativecommons.org/licenses/by/4.0/).

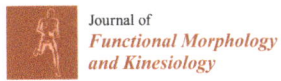

Journal of
Functional Morphology and Kinesiology

Article

Body Fat Assessment in International Elite Soccer Referees

Cristian Petri [1], Francesco Campa [2], Vitor Hugo Teixeira [3,4], Pascal Izzicupo [5], Giorgio Galanti [1], Angelo Pizzi [6], Georgian Badicu [7,*] and Gabriele Mascherini [1]

1. Sports and Exercise Medicine Unit, Clinical and Experimental Department, University of Florence, 50121 Firenze, Italy; cristian.petri@unifi.it (C.P.); giorgio.galanti@unifi.it (G.G.); gabriele.mascherini@unifi.it (G.M.)
2. Department for Life Quality Studies, University of Bologna, 47921 Rimini, Italy; francesco.campa3@unibo.it
3. Faculty of Nutrition and Food Sciences (FCNA), University of Porto, 4200-465 Porto, Portugal; vhugoteixeira@fcna.up.pt
4. Research Centre in Physical Activity, Health and Leisure (CIAFEL), Faculty of Sports, University of Porto, 4099-002 Porto, Portugal
5. Department of Medicine and Aging Science, "G. D'Annunzio" University of Chieti-Pescara, 66100 Chieti, Italy; pascalizzicupo@gmail.com
6. A.I.A., Italian Referees Association, 00187 Rome, Italy; angelopizzi@alice.it
7. Department of Physical Education and Special Motricity, Transilvania University of Brasov, 500068 Brasov, Romania
* Correspondence: georgian.badicu@unitbv.ro

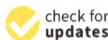

Received: 14 April 2020; Accepted: 5 June 2020; Published: 6 June 2020

Abstract: Soccer referees are a specific group in the sports population that are receiving increasing attention from sports scientists. A lower fat mass percentage (FM%) is a useful parameter to monitor fitness status and aerobic performance, while being able to evaluate it with a simple and quick field-based method can allow a regular assessment. The aim of this study was to provide a specific profile for referees based on morphological and body composition features while comparing the accuracy of different skinfold-based equations in estimating FM% in a cohort of soccer referees. Forty-three elite international soccer referees (age 38.8 ± 3.6 years), who participated in the 2018 Russian World Cup, underwent body composition assessments with skinfold thickness and dual-energy X-ray absorptiometry (DXA). Six equations used to derive FM% from skinfold thickness were compared with DXA measurements. The percentage of body fat estimated using DXA was 18.2 ± 4.1%, whereas skinfold-based FM% assessed from the six formulas ranged between 11.0% ± 1.7% to 15.6% ± 2.4%. Among the six equations considered, the Faulkner's formula showed the highest correlation with FM% estimated by DXA (r = 0.77; R^2 = 0.59 $p < 0.001$). Additionally, a new skinfold-based equation was developed: FM% = 8.386 + (0.478 × iliac crest skinfold) + (0.395 × abdominal skinfold, r = 0.78; R^2 = 0.61; standard error of the estimate (SEE) = 2.62 %; $p < 0.001$). Due to these findings, national and international federations will now be able to perform regular body composition assessments using skinfold measurements.

Keywords: anthropometry; body composition; DXA; equation; fat mass; soccer; somatotype; skinfolds

1. Introduction

No matter the competition level, there is no official soccer game without the presence of the 23rd key element: the referee. There are more than 840,000 registered referees who arbitrate soccer games each week verifying and enforcing the rules of the game [1]. However, scientific literature on referees in relation to physiological demands, body composition, and nutrition-related aspects [2–4] is limited when compared to what is available on players.

Not only do elite-class soccer referees need to perform their best in perceptual-cognitive abilities and decision-making tasks [5], but they must also achieve an elevated aerobic performance similar to a midfield soccer player [6]. Although there are significant differences between games, referees cover on average a distance between 9 and 13 km per game, depending on the level of competition [3,7–9]. Due to the high-intensity matches in recent years [10] and as a consequence of the increase in physical demand there is a trend towards a decrease in body mass index (BMI) and body fat levels in elite referees [11]. In fact, recent studies on elite referees (FIFA) show lower levels of BMI and body fat than previously reported in Premier League referees [12,13].

In soccer players, body fat is generally estimated by skinfold thickness assessment, bioelectrical impedance analysis, and dual-energy X-ray absorptiometry (DXA). DXA is widely accepted as a practical method for assessing fat mass in athletes [14–16] and is becoming more popular in elite sports as an analysis used by both practitioners and researchers [17]. Anthropometric assessment is another popular method used to predict body fat in athletes [18–20]. The measurement of skinfolds is widely adopted to monitor changes in body composition due to training and/or dietary interventions. Skinfold thickness measurements have long been utilized to predict body fat and over the years multiple equations have been developed for this purpose [21–26]. However, to the best of the authors' knowledge, there are no studies comparing results obtained by skinfold-based measurements and DXA in soccer referees.

This study was designed to present body composition features of soccer referees called for the Russian World Cup in 2018 with two main aims. The first purpose was to compare different equations to estimate fat mass from skinfold assessment with data derived from DXA. The second aim was to develop a prediction equation for estimating the percentage of fat mass (FM%) based on anthropometric variables specific for this cohort.

2. Materials and Methods

2.1. Study Population

Using a cross-sectional design, 43 elite international soccer referees (age 38.8 ± 3.6 years) from 6 confederations were enrolled in the study during a seminar held in the Federal Technical Center of Coverciano (Italy) in April 2018, during the competitive season. They were classified as elite because they were either registered at the maximum level in the athletic federation or have received financial support for their dedication to training and games. The study was designed and conducted in accordance with the Helsinki Declaration. The ethics committee of the Italian football association approved this study and all the participants signed written informed consent prior to their inclusion in the study (approval code: 03032018).

2.2. Procedures

Participants underwent body composition assessments early in the morning, in an overnight-fasted state, and at least 12 h postexercise, with no long trips during the previous day. Further, the consumption of alcohol and stimulant beverages were not allowed for at least 15 h prior to testing.

The methodology used for the assessment of body composition was in accordance with our previous studies [26,27], using the integration of anthropometry, skinfold thickness, and DXA. Anthropometric measurements were taken following the protocol of The International Society for the Advancement of Kinanthropometry (ISAK) [28] by the same researcher (an ISAK level anthropometrist), whose technical error was 5% and 1.5% for skinfolds and all other measurements, respectively. Height (m) and body weight (kg) were measured to the nearest 0.1 cm and 0.01 kg, respectively, using a high-precision mechanical scale (SECA, Basel, Switzerland). BMI was calculated using the formula body mass/height^2 (kg/m^2). Biceps girth, waist girth, and hip girth (cm) were measured with a narrow, metallic, and inextensible measuring tape (Lufkin® model W606PM, London, UK; precision = 1 mm). Skinfolds were measured with a skinfold caliper (Holtain Ltd., Crymych, UK; precision = 0.2 mm) at nine anatomical sites (triceps, subscapular, biceps, iliac crest, supraspinal, pectoral, abdominal, thigh, and calf). Humerus and femur breadths were measured to the nearest 0.1 cm with a sliding caliper (GMP, Zürich, Switzerland). Somatotype was calculated according to the Heath-Carter method [29].

Body density was calculated from the Siri equation [30] adapted for age [31], which was then used to estimate FM%. The following six skinfold-based equations were used to estimate FM%:

- Yushaz [21];
- Faulkner [22];
- Eston et al. [24];
- Durnin and Womersley [23];
- Reilly et al. [25];
- Suarez et al. [26].

Additionally, the average FM% measured by all of these equations was considered. Fat-Free Mass (FFM) was calculated subtracting fat mass from body weight.

A DXA scanner (Hologic QDR Series, Delphi A model, Bedford, MA, USA) with Hologic APEX 13.3:3 software version, was used to estimate FM%. The instrument was calibrated with phantoms as per the manufacturer's guidelines each day prior to measurements. Participants assumed a stationary supine position on the scanning table. All scanning and analyses were performed by the same technician to ensure consistency and in accordance with standardized testing protocols recognized as best practice [17,32,33].

2.3. Statistical Analysis

Data were expressed as mean ± standard deviations (SD) and normality of distribution of the data was verified by the Kolmogorov–Smirnov test. Comparisons between FM% calculated with the different formulas and those measured by DXA were made using linear regression analysis, as well as between the sum of skinfold measurements with FM% obtained by DXA.

Given the fact that different ethnic groups participated, the effect of ethnicity on FM% was tested using the Kruskal–Wallis test. No interactions were found between ethnicity and other independent variables; therefore, we used the whole sample in the model development. The ability of the following variables (age, stature, weight, and skinfolds) in predicting FM% in the international soccer referees was assessed using stepwise regression analysis. During model development, normality of residuals and homogeneity of variance were tested. Significance at $p \leq 0.05$ was established as the criterion for inclusion of a predictor whereas removal criteria were set at $p \leq 0.1$. If more than one variable remained in the model, and to assess multicollinearity, a variance inflation factor (threshold as 5) was calculated for each independent variable. The data were analyzed using the statistical package IBM SPSS Statistics (version 13.0) for Windows. (SPSS Inc., Chicago, IL, USA).

3. Results

General and anthropometric characteristics and descriptive values of FM% estimated from DXA and skinfold-based equations are shown in Table 1. The referees showed an average balanced mesomorph somatotype, characterized by a dominant mesomorph component and similar values between endomorph and ectomorph components (no more than a difference of 0.5 units, Figure 1).

Correlation coefficients and level of significant differences between FM% with DXA and other practical estimates in the soccer referees are shown in Table 2. Given that no difference between ethnic groups in FM% was found ($p = 0.241$), all the values were presented together.

Table 1. General and anthropometric characteristics of the international-level elite referees.

Variable	Mean	SD	Minimum	Maximum
Age (year)	38.8	3.6	29.5	44.1
Body Mass (kg)	75.7	6.5	61.0	94.0
Height (m)	1.8	0.1	1.7	1.9
Body mass index (kg/m^2)	23.1	1.3	20.6	25.8
Endomorphy	2.7	0.9	1.2	5.1
Mesomorphy	6.5	1.2	4.2	8.5
Ectomorphy	2.9	0.7	1.2	4.6
Fat Mass by DXA (%)	18.2	4.1	11.5	28.0
Fat Mass by Eston et al. [24] (%)	12.0	2.4	9.4	18.8
Fat Mass by Yuhasz [21] (%)	12.8	2.5	8.8	21.0
Fat Mass by Faulkner [22] (%)	12.7	2.1	9.2	18.5
Fat Mass by Reilly et al. [25] (%)	11.0	1.7	8.2	16.5
Fat Mass by Suarez et al. [26] (%)	15.6	2.4	12.6	24.6
Fat Mass by Durnin and Womersley [23] (%)	13.3	2.9	8.5	20.5
Fat Mass by Mean (%)	12.9	2.2	9.7	19.4
Σ2sk (mm)	14.1	5.0	7.8	29.6
Σ4sk-a (mm)	32.4	8.5	21.0	57.3
Σ4sk-b (mm)	38.6	11.4	21.6	75.6
Σ5sk (mm)	41.7	10.7	27.9	74.5
Σ6sk (mm)	59.6	16.4	34.0	112.6
Σ7sk (mm)	62.9	16.6	38.9	116.8
Σ9sk (mm)	73.7	18.2	46.5	130.8

Abbreviations: Σ2sk = anterior thigh, medial calf; Σ4sk-a = biceps, triceps, subscapular, iliac crest; Σ4sk-b = triceps, abdominal; anterior thigh, medial calf; Σ5sk = biceps, triceps, subscapular, iliac crest, anterior thigh; Σ6sk = triceps, subscapular, iliac crest, abdominal, anterior thigh, medial calf; Σ7sk = triceps, subscapular, iliac crest, supraspinal, abdominal, anterior thigh, medial calf; Σ9sk = biceps, triceps, subscapular, iliac crest, supraspinal, pectoral, abdominal, anterior thigh, medial calf.

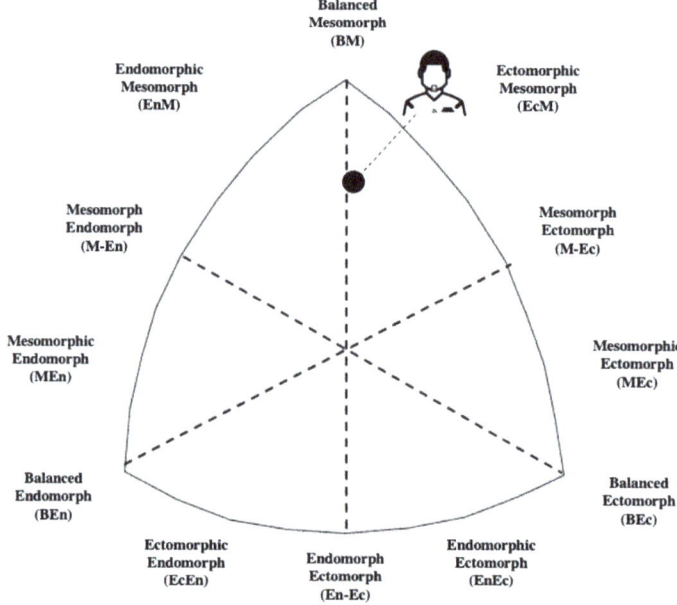

Figure 1. Representation of the somatotype of the International elite male soccer referees.

Table 2. Correlation coefficients and level of significance between fat mass percentage (FM%) estimated by dual-energy X-ray absorptiometry (DXA) with the sum of skinfold measurements, and FM% obtained from skinfold-based equations.

Variable	r	R^2	p-Value
$\sum 2sk$	0.41	0.165	0.007
$\sum 4sk$	0.75	0.559	<0.001
$\sum 4sk$	0.70	0.491	<0.001
$\sum 5sk$	0.72	0.519	<0.001
$\sum 6sk$	0.76	0.585	<0.001
$\sum 7sk$	0.77	0.588	<0.001
$\sum 9sk$	0.76	0.581	<0.001
Fat Mass by Eston et al. [24]	0.60	0.363	<0.001
Fat Mass by Yuhasz [21]	0.76	0.585	<0.001
Fat Mass by Faulkner [22]	0.77	0.598	<0.001
Fat Mass by Reilly et al. [25]	0.71	0.497	<0.001
Fat Mass by Suarez et al. [26]	0.74	0.549	<0.001
Fat Mass by Durnin and Womersley [23]	0.76	0.580	<0.001
Fat Mass by Mean	0.78	0.606	<0.001

All FM% values obtained by the skinfold-based equations showed large to very large positive correlations (r from 0.60 to 0.78) to those measured by DXA. The FM% estimated from all of the equations showed significant differences ($p < 0.001$) in comparison to the DXA results. The sum of skinfold measurements showed moderate to very large positive correlations with FM% obtained by DXA, except for the sum of two skinfold measurements. Relationships between DXA-derived FM% and skinfold thicknesses of different anatomical sites are shown in Table 3. The vast majority of skinfold measurements cited showed moderate to very large positive relationships with FM% (r from 0.57 to 0.71), except biceps, pectoral, anterior thigh, and medial calf.

Table 3. Relationships between DXA-derived FM% and different skinfolds measured in the international-level elite referees.

Variable	r	R^2	p-Value
Biceps	0.25	0.060	0.113
Triceps	0.57	0.321	<0.001
Subscapular	0.63	0.394	<0.001
Iliac crest	0.71	0.510	<0.001
Supraspinal	0.53	0.285	<0.001
Pectoral	0.02	0.001	0.885
Abdominal	0.68	0.464	<0.001
Anterior thigh	0.37	0.135	0.016
Medial calf	0.39	0.154	0.009
BMI	0.10	0.011	0.505

Table 4 shows the skinfold-based model for FM% generated for the international soccer referees. Only variables contributing as significant predictors using backward stepwise approach were used in the model. The final prediction model included: FM% = 8.386 + (0.478 × iliac crest skinfold) + (0.395 × abdominal skinfold, r = 0.781; R^2 = 0.610; SEE = 2.62 %; $p < 0.001$, Table 4; Figure 2).

Table 4. Developed models for FM% prediction.

Variable	Coefficient	R^2	SEE (%)
Model 1		0.510	2.90
Intercept	9.727		
Iliac crest skinfold (mm)	0.714		
Model 2		0.610	2.62
Intercept	8.386		
Iliac crest skinfold (mm)	0.478		
Abdominal skinfold (mm)	0.395		

Abbreviations: R^2, coefficient of determination; SEE, standard error of the estimate.

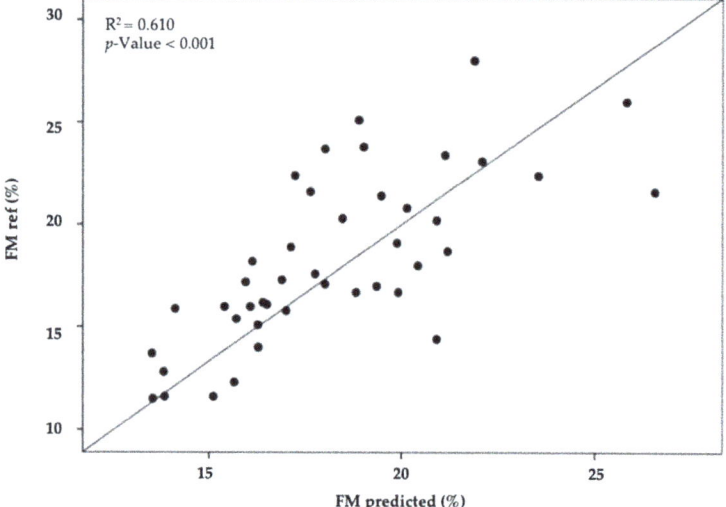

Figure 2. The scatter plot illustrates the results of the regression analysis for FM% obtained by the reference method (DXA) and predicted by the equation developed in the sample of international soccer referees.

4. Discussion

This study compared six skinfold-based equations showing the different results in FM% estimation in international elite soccer referees, using DXA as a reference method. Additionally, our study is the first to have provided a specific equation for this particular sample group, as well as descriptive body composition parameters. Our results highlight that the sum of skinfold thickness measurements taken in seven (triceps, subscapular, iliac crest, supraspinal, abdominal, anterior thigh, and medial calf) or in nine (biceps, triceps, subscapular, iliac crest, supraspinal, pectoral, abdominal, anterior thigh, and medial calf) sites show a high association with the FM% estimated with DXA. Secondly, among the equations considered, that of Faulkner [22] showed the best sensitivity in assessing FM% in the international elite soccer referees. Lastly, a new equation based on the anthropometric measurements taken on the sample group was proposed.

While excessive FM% may affect performance, body composition is an aspect of considerable interest to scientists, athletes, and coaches [34]. Typical FM% values (ranging from 5% to 19%) reported in male athletes depends on the sport, playing position, and methodology used for the assessment [35–37]. In particular, male soccer players show a percentage of fat mass ranging between 11.7–13.7% [20,38]. Furthermore, the tested referees in this study showed a balanced mesomorph somatotype.

Similarly, high-level soccer players are characterized by a balanced mesomorph morphology but their somatotype can also be endomorphic mesomorph, ectomorphic mesomorph, mesomorph ectomoprh, and mesomorphic ectomorph [39]; in all these cases, the dominant component is the mesomorphy, but there is a different balance between endomorphy and ectomorphy, probably due to the different roles of the game.

Our results showed substantial discrepancies in FM% prediction depending on the method plied. Therefore, care must be taken when feedback on FM% is provided to soccer referees since values are likely to be method dependent. With the exception of FM% obtained using Suarez's equation [26] or estimated by DXA, most of the data found was within the range described in the literature. As opposed to Faulkner's equation [22], the new formula suggested appears to be a simpler and faster alternative as it is specific to soccer referees. Furthermore, the use of only two skinfold sites, provides an advantage in the field-based assessment of FM%, representing a more efficient use of time.

Contrary to previous studies of elite soccer players [25,26], data collected in the present study showed that measurements of the lower body skinfolds are not accurate when predicting FM%. In this study, thigh skinfold thickness was not entered in the developed model representing strength in the new formula because it has been acknowledged that the anterior thigh skinfold is one of the least accurate sites to measure [23,24]. Furthermore, our results showed that different sums of skinfolds measured on the referees showed moderate to large correlations with DXA data, used as a criterion method. The results of the present study showed very large correlations between Σ4SKF-a, Σ4SKF-b, Σ6SKF, Σ7SKF, and Σ9SKF with FM% estimated by DXA, similar to the associations with the data found in the literature for elite soccer players [40,41]. Thus, considering the substantial differences observed between the different equations and their similar and/or lower correlations with the DXA-derived FM%, even the sum of skinfold measurements appears to be a good alternative approach in obtaining information on body fat distribution in elite soccer referees.

Some of the strengths in this study include the selection of international-level male soccer referees, all with experience in international matches. Skinfold measurement is a practical, low cost, and easily accessible alternative to more complex and expensive methods such as DXA. Consequently, the present study provides a noninvasive, cost-free, and fast tool to accurately estimate FM% in the investigated cohort. Moreover, the DXA method might not be feasible or useful when financial resources are limited or when a whole group is repeatedly measured, because up to 10 min for each person is required.

However, the use of DXA as a reference method poses some limitations in the development and comparison of new equations for assessing fat mass. Most of the equations in the literature are based on the reference of hydrostatic weighing. This could predispose our equation to an overestimation of body fat. Additional limitations regarding sample size should be addressed. The sample consisted exclusively of male subjects thus, further studies involving elite female referees are needed. Furthermore, the lack of a validation sample did not allow the test of the performance of the new equation at a group level (e.g., analysis of the regression coefficients, line of identity, R^2, RMSE) and at the individual level using the Bland–Altman analysis.

The practical application of this equation facilitates an increasingly accurate evaluation of the athlete. The soccer referee can be considered in all respects as an athlete, even sports research has deepened this particular population. First, the components of the physical load required during a competition [3,7,9] have been evaluated, more recently the nutritional aspects have had an increase in interest [4,12,42,43]. In this context of energy balance, the development of a new equation for the evaluation of the fat mass with a specific reference to the analyzed population allows a more accurate, reliable, and repeatable evaluation during the competitive season of the soccer referee through a field methodology.

5. Conclusions

All the equations investigated (Eston et al. [24], Yuhasz [21], Reilly et al. [25], Suarez et al. [26], and Durnin and Womersley [23]) showed positive correlations in comparison with DXA data. In particular, the equations developed by Faulkner [22] showed the best sensitivity in assessing FM% compared to DXA. Additionally, the sum of seven skinfolds, which included triceps, subscapular, iliac crest, supraspinal, abdominal, anterior thigh, and medial calf measurements showed a high correlation with FM% measured by DXA, representing an alternative approach in body composition assessment. Finally, this study provides a new formula for FM% estimation in international-level male soccer referees [FM% = 8.386 + (0.478 × iliac crest skinfold) + (0.395 × abdominal skinfold)].

Author Contributions: Conceptualization, C.P. and G.M. methodology, C.P., F.C., and P.I.; formal analysis, C.P., F.C., and P.I.; investigation, A.P., G.G., and C.P.; data curation, C.P., F.C., and P.I.; writing—original draft preparation, V.H.T., C.P., and G.B.; visualization, G.B., V.H.T., and G.M.; supervision, F.C., G.B., and G.M. All authors have read and agreed to the published version of the manuscript.

Funding: This research received no external funding.

Acknowledgments: The authors gratefully acknowledge FIFA for their support of this research during the experiments.

Conflicts of Interest: The authors declare no conflicts of interest.

References

1. FIFA Big Count 2006. Available online: http://www.fifa.com/mm/document/fifafacts/bcoffsurv/bigcount.statspackage_7024.pdf (accessed on 14 March 2019).
2. Caballero, J.A.R.; Ojeda, E.B.; Sarmiento, S.; Valdivielso, M.N.; García-Manso, J.M.; García-Aranda, J.M.; Mallo, J.; Helsen, W. Physiological profile of national-level Spanish soccer referees. *Int. Sportmed. J.* **2011**, *51*, 633–638.
3. Weston, M.; Castagna, C.; Impellizzeri, F.M.; Bizzini, M.; Williams, A.M.; Gregson, W. Science and medicine applied to soccer refereeing: An update. *Sports Med.* **2012**, *42*, 615–631. [CrossRef] [PubMed]
4. Teixeira, V.H.; Gonçalves, L.; Meneses, T.; Moreira, P. Nutritional intake of elite football referees. *J. Sports Sci.* **2014**, *32*, 1279–1285. [CrossRef]
5. Helsen, W.; Bultynck, J.B. Physical and perceptual-cognitive demands of top-class refereeing in association football. *J. Sports Sci.* **2004**, *22*, 179–189. [CrossRef]
6. Bizzini, M.; Junge, A.; Bahr, R.; Dvorak, J. Female soccer referees selected for the FIFA Women's World Cup 2007: Survey of injuries and musculoskeletal problems. *Br. J. Sports Med.* **2009**, *43*, 936–942. [CrossRef] [PubMed]
7. Krustrup, P.; Helsen, W.; Randers, M.B.; Christensen, J.F.; Macdonald, C.; Rebelo, A.N.; Bangsbo, J. Activity profile and physical demands of football referees and assistant referees in international games. *J. Sports Sci.* **2009**, *27*, 1167–1176. [CrossRef] [PubMed]
8. Mallo, J.; Veiga, S.; Lopez de Subijana, C.; Navarro, E. Activity profile of top-class female soccer refereeing in relation to the position of the ball. *J. Sci. Med. Sport* **2010**, *13*, 129–132. [CrossRef]
9. Weston, M.; Drust, B.; Gregson, W. Intensities of exercise during match-play in FA Premier League referees and players. *J. Sports Sci.* **2011**, *29*, 527–532. [CrossRef]
10. Barnes, C.; Archer, D.T.; Hogg, B.; Bush, M.; Bradley, P.S. The evolution of physical and technical performance parameters in the English Premier League. *Int. J. Sports Med.* **2014**, *35*, 1095–1100. [CrossRef]
11. Casajús, J.A.; Gonzalez-Aguero, A. Body composition evolution in elite referees; an eleven-years retrospective study. *Int. J. Sports Med.* **2015**, *36*, 550–553. [CrossRef]
12. Schenk, K.; Bizzini, M.; Gatterer, H. Exercise physiology and nutritional perspectives of elite soccer referee ing. *Scand. J. Med. Sci. Sports* **2018**, *28*, 782–793. [CrossRef] [PubMed]
13. Reilly, T.; Gregson, W. Special populations: The referee and assistant referee. *J. Sports Sci.* **2006**, *24*, 795–801. [CrossRef] [PubMed]
14. Campa, F.; Matias, C.N.; Marini, E.; Heymsfield, S.B.; Toselli, S.; Sardinha, L.B.; Silva, A.M. Identifying Athlete Body Fluid Changes During a Competitive Season With Bioelectrical Impedance Vector Analysis. *Int. J. Sports Physiol. Perform.* **2020**, *15*, 361–367. [CrossRef] [PubMed]
15. Marini, E.; Campa, F.; Toselli, S.; Stagi, S.; Matias, C.N.; Toselli, S.; Sardinha, L.B.; Silva, A.M. Phase Angle and Bioelectrical Impedance Vector Analysis in the Evaluation of Body Composition in Athletes. *Clin. Nutr.* **2020**, *39*, 447–454. [CrossRef]
16. Núñez, J.; Diego, M.I.; Suárez-Arrones, L. Validity of Field Methods to Estimate Fat-Free Mass Changes Throughout the Season in Elite Youth Soccer Players. *Front. Physiol.* **2020**, *11*, 16. [CrossRef]

17. Milsom, J.; Naughton, R.; O'Boyle, A.; Iqbal, Z.; Morgans, R.; Drust, B.; Morton, J.P. Body composition assessment of English premier league soccer players: A comparative DXA analysis of first team, U21 and U18 squads. *J. Sports Sci.* **2015**, *33*, 1799–1806. [CrossRef]
18. Toselli, S.; Campa, F. Anthropometry and Functional Movement Patterns in Elite Male Volleyball Players of Different Competitive Levels. *J. Strength Cond. Res.* **2018**, *32*, 2601–2611. [CrossRef]
19. Campa, F.; Semprini, G.; Júdice, P.B.; Messina, G.; Toselli, S. Anthropometry, Physical and Movement Features, and Repeated-sprint Ability in Soccer Players. *Int. J. Sports Med.* **2019**, *40*, 100–109. [CrossRef]
20. Campa, F.; Piras, A.; Raffi, M.; Toselli, S. Functional Movement Patterns and Body Composition of High-Level Volleyball, Soccer, and Rugby Players. *J. Sport Rehabil.* **2019**, *28*, 740–745. [CrossRef]
21. Yuhasz, M.S. *The Effects of Sports Training on Body Fat in Man with Predictions of Optimal Body Weight*; University of Illinois at Urbana-Champaign: Urbana, IL, USA, 1962.
22. Faulkner, J.A. *Physiology of Swimming and Diving*; Baltimore Academic Press: New York, NY, USA, 1968; pp. 415–446.
23. Durnin, J.V.; Womersley, J. Body fat assessed from total body density and its estimation from skinfold thickness: Measurements on 481 men and women aged from 16 to 72 years. *Br. J. Nutr.* **1974**, *32*, 77–97. [CrossRef]
24. Eston, R.G.; Rowlands, A.V.; Charlesworth, S.; Davies, A.; Hoppitt, T. Prediction of DXA-determined whole body fat from skinfolds: Importance of including skinfolds from the thigh and calf in young, healthy men and women. *Eur. J. Clin. Nutr.* **2005**, *59*, 695–702. [CrossRef] [PubMed]
25. Reilly, T.; George, K.; Marfell-Jones, M.; Scott, M.; Sutton, L.; Wallace, J.A. How well do skinfold equations predict percent body fat in elite soccer players? *Int. J. Sports Med.* **2009**, *30*, 607–613. [CrossRef] [PubMed]
26. Suarez-Arrones, L.; Petri, C.; Maldonado, R.A.; Torreno, N.; Munguía-Izquierdo, D.; Di Salvo, V.; Méndez-Villanueva, A. Body fat assessment in elite soccer players: Cross-validation of different field methods. *Sci. Med. Footb.* **2018**, *2*, 203–208. [CrossRef]
27. Mascherini, G.; Petri, C.; Galanti, G. Integrated total body composition and localized fat-free mass assessment. *Sport Sci. Health* **2015**, *11*, 217–225. [CrossRef]
28. Steward, A.; Marfell-Jones, M. *International Standards for Anthropometric Assessment*; International Society for the Advancement of Kinanthropometry: Lower Hutt, New Zealand, 2014.
29. Carter, J.E.L. *The Heath-Carter Anthropometric Somatotype*; San Diego State University: San Diego, CA, USA, 2002.
30. Siri, W.E. The gross composition of the body. *Adv. Biol. Med. Phys.* **1956**, *4*, 239–280. [PubMed]
31. Wells, J.C.K. *The Evolutionary Biology of Human Body Fatness: Thrift and Control*; Cambridge University Press: Cambridge, UK, 2009.
32. Rodriguez-Sanchez, N.; Galloway, S.D. Errors in dual energy x-ray absorptiometry estimation of body composition induced by hypohydration. *Int. J. Sport Nutr. Exerc. Metab.* **2015**, *25*, 60–68. [CrossRef] [PubMed]
33. Nana, A.; Slater, G.J.; Hopkins, W.G.; Halson, S.L.; Martin, D.T.; West, N.P.; Burke, L.M. Importance of standardized DXA protocol for assessing physique changes in athletes. *Int. J. Sport Nutr. Exerc. Metab.* **2016**, *26*, 259–267. [CrossRef]
34. Malina, R.M. Body composition in athletes: Assessment and estimated fatness. *Clin. Sports Med.* **2007**, *26*, 37–68. [CrossRef]
35. Campa, F.; Matias, C.; Gatterer, H.; Toselli, S.; Koury, J.C.; Andreoli, A.; Melchiorri, G.; Sardinha, L.B.; Silva, A.M. Classic Bioelectrical Impedance Vector Reference Values for Assessing Body Composition in Male and Female Athletes. *Int. J. Environ. Res. Public Health* **2019**, *16*, 5066. [CrossRef]
36. Campa, F.; Toselli, S. Bioimpedance Vector Analysis of Elite, Subelite, and Low-Level Male Volleyball Players. *Int. J. Sports Physiol. Perform.* **2018**, *13*, 1250–1253. [CrossRef]
37. Jeukendrup, A.; Gleeson, M. *Sport Nutrition: An Introduction to Energy Production and Performance*; Human Kinetics Publishers: Champaign, IL, USA, 2010.
38. Campa, F.; Silva, A.M.; Iannuzzi, V.; Mascherini, G.; Benedetti, L.; Toselli, S. The role of somatic maturation on bioimpedance patterns and body composition in male elite youth soccer players. *Int. J. Environ. Res. Public Health* **2019**, *16*, 4711. [CrossRef] [PubMed]
39. Campa, F.; Silva, A.M.; Talluri, J.; Matias, C.N.; Badicu, G.; Toselli, S. Somatotype and Bioimpedance Vector Analysis: A New Target Zone for Male Athletes. *Sustainability* **2020**, *12*, 4365. [CrossRef]

40. Garrido-Chamorro, R.; Sirvent-Belando, J.E.; González-Lorenzo, M.; Blasco-Lafarga, C.; Roche, E. Skinfold sum: Reference values for top athletes. *Int. J. Morphol.* **2012**, *30*, 803–809. [CrossRef]
41. Santos, D.A.; Dawson, J.A.; Matias, C.N.; Rocha, P.M.; Minderico, C.S. Reference Values for Body Composition and Anthropometric Measurements in Athletes. *PLoS ONE* **2014**, *9*, 97846. [CrossRef] [PubMed]
42. Mascherini, G.; Petri, C.; Ermini, E.; Pizzi, A.; Ventura, A.; Galanti, G. Eating Habits and Body Composition of International Elite Soccer Referees. *J. Hum. Kinet.* **2020**, *71*, 145–153. [CrossRef]
43. Campa, F.; Piras, A.; Raffi, M.; Trofè, A.; Perazzolo, M.; Mascherini, G.; Toselli, S. The Effects of Dehydration on Metabolic and Neuromuscular Functionality during Cycling. *Int. J. Environ. Res. Public Health* **2020**, *17*, 1161. [CrossRef] [PubMed]

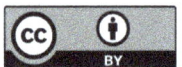

© 2020 by the authors. Licensee MDPI, Basel, Switzerland. This article is an open access article distributed under the terms and conditions of the Creative Commons Attribution (CC BY) license (http://creativecommons.org/licenses/by/4.0/).

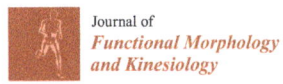

Article

Potential Use of Wearable Sensors to Assess Cumulative Kidney Trauma in Endurance Off-Road Running

Daniel Rojas-Valverde [1,2,*], Rafael Timón [2], Braulio Sánchez-Ureña [3], José Pino-Ortega [4], Ismael Martínez-Guardado [2] and Guillermo Olcina [2,*]

1. Centro de Investigación y Diagnóstico en Salud y Deporte (CIDISAD), Escuela Ciencias del Movimiento Humano y Calidad de Vida (CIEMHCAVI), Universidad Nacional, Heredia 86-3000, Costa Rica
2. Grupo en Avances en el Entrenamiento Deportivo y Acondicionamiento Físico (GAEDAF), Facultad Ciencias del Deporte, Universidad de Extremadura, 10005 Cáceres, Spain; rtimon@unex.es (R.T.); wismi4@gmail.com (I.M.-G.)
3. Programa Ciencias del Ejercicio y la Salud (PROCESA), Escuela Ciencias del Movimiento Humano y Calidad de Vida (CIEMHCAVI), Universidad Nacional, Heredia 86-3000, Costa Rica; brau09@hotmail.com
4. Departmento de Actividad Física y Deporte, Facultad Ciencias del Deporte, 30720 Murcia, Spain; josepinoortega@um.es
* Correspondence: drojasv@hotmail.com (D.R.-V.); golcina@unex.es (G.O.); Tel.: +506-88250219 (D.R.-V.)

Received: 6 November 2020; Accepted: 11 December 2020; Published: 14 December 2020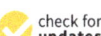

Abstract: (1) Background: This study aimed to explore wearable sensors' potential use to assess cumulative mechanical kidney trauma during endurance off-road running. (2) Methods: 18 participants (38.78 ± 10.38 years, 73.24 ± 12.6 kg, 172.17 ± 9.48 cm) ran 36 k off-road race wearing a Magnetic, Angular Rate and Gravity (MARG) sensor attached to their lower back. Impacts in g forces were recorded throughout the race using the MARG sensor. Two blood samples were collected immediately pre- and post-race: serum creatinine (sCr) and albumin (sALB). (3) Results: Sixteen impact variables were grouped using principal component analysis in four different principal components (PC) that explained 90% of the total variance. The 4th PC predicted 24% of the percentage of change (∆%) of sCr and the 3rd PC predicted the ∆% of sALB by 23%. There were pre- and post-race large changes in sCr and sALB ($p \leq 0.01$) and 33% of participants met acute kidney injury diagnosis criteria. (4) Conclusions: The data related to impacts could better explain the cumulative mechanical kidney trauma during mountain running, opening a new range of possibilities using technology to better understand how the number and magnitude of the g-forces involved in off-road running could potentially affect kidney function.

Keywords: renal health; wearable devices; technology; acute kidney injury; inertial measurement units (IMU)

---

1. Introduction

Acute kidney injury (AKI) is a relatively uncommon condition in sports. This condition has been reported in prolonged and repetitive strenuous exercises [1]. It is understood as a transitional decrease in renal function, expressed by a reduction in glomerular filtration rate, increase in serum creatinine (sCr) and albumin (sALB), and alterations of other novel AKI-related urine and blood biomarkers during a relatively short period (1–3 days) [2].

The evidence of AKI cases in both contact and non-contact sports has been increased, but with clear different etiological backgrounds [3–5]. In contact sports like football, boxing, and rugby, AKI cases have been related to kidney contusion or trauma (grade I in American Association for Surgery of

Trauma classification) during tackles, punches, or other high-intensity actions with direct impact to the body [6,7]. On the other hand, in non-contact sports (e.g., endurance running and cycling), AKI has been related to the high number of muscle eccentric-concentric contractions leading to muscle damage [8,9].

In endurance running and mainly off-road running [8,10], some evidence has been published regarding the impact of external workload (e.g., impacts) as an additional factor that may contribute to AKI incidence, next to other known factors like dehydration, heat strain, and high metabolic activity [11]. Within this multifactorial etiology, high physical internal and external load seems to be a discernible contributing factor to the transitory decrease in renal function in endurance runners [12]. It could be due to muscle damage in response to high eccentric actions and its effect on inflammatory and hemodynamic responses that may affect the kidney [13]. New evidence has also highlighted the cumulative mechanical trauma that affects the kidney during off-road running as a potential cause of AKI [9]. Although kidneys are very well protected structures, there is relative mobility that could lead to injury even when no direct trauma occurred [14], for example, during downhill running or change of directions during training or competition.

Monitoring physical load is critical in endurance sports, such as off-road running, due to the high number of actions involved [15]. This is why non-invasive tools as wearable sensors could be an accessible option to assess potential cumulative mechanical kidney trauma, indirectly analyzing the mobility of anatomical structures near the kidneys, such as the lower back. These wearable sensors are used to monitor physical load during exercise in different parts of the body, such as the wrist, waist, and trunk [16–18]. It has also been determined that there is a relationship between the increase in serum blood factors related to kidney damage and the quantified load in the lower back [9]. Therefore, this study aimed to explore the potential use of wearable Magnetic, Angular Rate and Gravity (MARG) sensors to assess cumulative mechanical kidney trauma during off-road running.

2. Materials and Methods

2.1. Design

Participants were asked to perform three loops of a 12 km (+ascend = 600 m) circuit (total distance = 36 km and total +ascend = 1800 m), under 25° Celsius of temperature, and 80% of humidity (Wet Bulb globe Temperature, 3M, USA). Runners wore a MARG sensor attached to the lower back during the race, and variables of time-related impacts were extracted. Two blood samples were collected pre- and post-race to assess serum creatinine (sCr) and albumin (sALB). An analysis was made to explore a model based on impact variables that explained sCr and sALB increases between pre- and post-race.

2.2. Participants

Eighteen experienced mountain runners participated in this study (age 38.78 ± 10.38 years, weight 73.24 ± 12.6 kg, height 172.17 ± 9.48 cm). They had 4.78 ± 2.42 years of experience competing in ultra-endurance events. Participant's mean finish time was 4.2 ± 0.21 h. No neuromuscular, metabolic, or structural injuries were reported at least six months before the study. The participants were asked to avoid intense endurance exercise at least a week before the event.

All participants were notified of the study's aim, protocol details and the potential risks and rights during their participation. The study's protocol followed all biomedical guidelines based on the Declaration of Helsinki (2013) and it was reviewed and approved by the Institutional Review Boards of Universidad Nacional (Reg. Code 2019-P005) and Universidad de Extremadura (Reg. Code 139/2020).

2.3. Materials and Procedures

Sixteen different time-related impacts (*n*/min, g forces) variables were assessed using a Magnetic, Angular Rate and Gravity (MARG) sensor (WIMU PRO™, RealTrack Systems, Almería, Spain). The devices were attached to the lower back (~L1–L3) [9] of each participant with a special spandex dark belt adjusted with elastic straps to avoid device's unwanted vibrations or movements (see Figure 1). The MARG's integrate four 3-axis microelectromechanical systems accelerometers (2x ± 16 g, 1x ± 32 g, and 1x ± 400 g), gyroscope, and magnetometer. All MARG's calibration and setting were developed following published guidelines [19,20], its reliability for neuromuscular running physical load assessment has been proven [21] and its reliability has been tested in different body parts [22]. The variables extracted were total impacts per min (Impacts$_{Total}$/min) and fifteen progressively scaled categories of g-force magnitude, each 1 g wide (Impacts$_{1-15\,g}$/min).

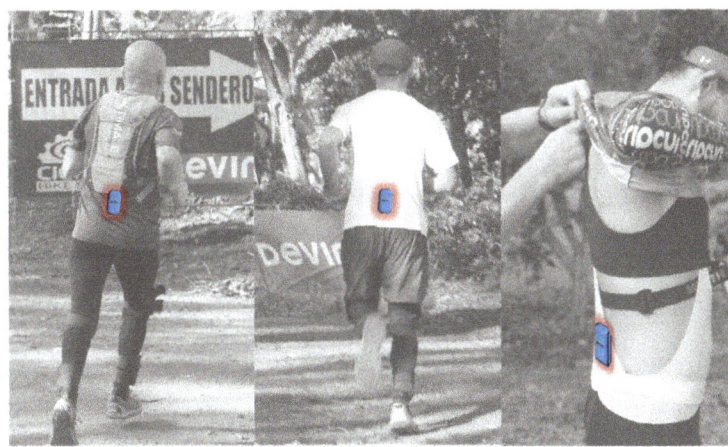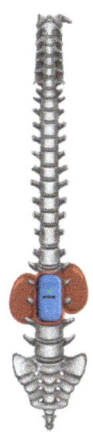

Figure 1. Inertial measurement unit attachment at runner's lower back (L1–L3).

Blood serum samples were collected using 5 mL blood spray-coated silica tubes (BD Vacutainer®, Franklin Lakes, NJ, USA). After centrifugation (10 min at 2000 g), samples were stored at −20 °C. After 24 h, the samples were processed by the photometry method using an automatic biochemical analyzer (BS-200E, Mindray, China). The variable analyzed was serum creatinine (sCr, mg/dL) and serum albumin (sALB, IU/L). Acute kidney injury (sCr baseline in mg/dL *1.5) was considered following established diagnosis criteria [23]. Two groups were made based on AKI diagnosis as follows: those participants that met AKI diagnosis (AKI) and the ones that did not (No-AKI), in order to explore differences in the number of impacts reported.

Urine specific gravity (USG) was assessed as a hydration status marker. USG was confirmed and double-checked with a digital valid [24] handheld refractometer (Palm AbbeTM, Misco, Solon, OH, USA). It was classified following the hydration status ranges: well-hydrated <1.01, minimal dehydration 1.01–1.02, significant dehydration 1.02–1.03, and severe dehydration >1.03 [25]. The refractometer was cleaned with distilled water and calibrated previously. There were no reported urination problems or difficulties neither before nor after the race.

2.4. Statistical Analysis

All sixteen impact variables were grouped using a Principal Component Analysis (PCA) following previous studies guidelines [9,26]. PCA was suitable, according to Kaiser-Meyer-Olkin ($KMO = 0.63$) values and the Barleth Sphericity test ($p < 0.01$). Eigenvalues (EV) > 1 were considered for the extraction of each Principal Component (PC). A VariMax-orthogonal rotation method was used to identify the high correlation of components. A threshold of 0.6 was set to retain loadings. The highest loading was used when a cross-loading was found between PCs. PCA procedure followed standard quality criteria [27], meeting 21 out of 21 of the quality items.

A paired t-test was used to explore sCr and sALB changes between pre- and post-race data and the Change delta's percentage (Δ%) was calculated as follows: ((sCr post-race–sCr pre-race)/sCr pre-race)*100. An unpaired t-test was performed to explore potential differences in the number of impacts between those participants who met AKI diagnosis and those who did not. USG data were analyzed using a repeated measure *t*-test. The magnitude of the differences was calculated using Cohen´s d.

Finally, a stepwise regression model (R^2) was applied to resulted factor scores obtained from impact´s PCA using the Δ% of sCr and sALB as the dependent variable. This statistical technique was applied to identify which impact´s PC could predict the Δ% of sCr, and Δ% of sALB.

All variables were presented in mean ± standard deviation. Alpha was set at $p < 0.05$ and all analyses were made using the Statistical Package for Social Science (v.22, SPSS, Chicago, IL, USA).

3. Results

Participants experienced a total of 170.57 ± 34.42 impacts per minute. Figure 2 shows the mean number of impacts per minute in relation to the associated magnitude of g-force (see Figure 2).

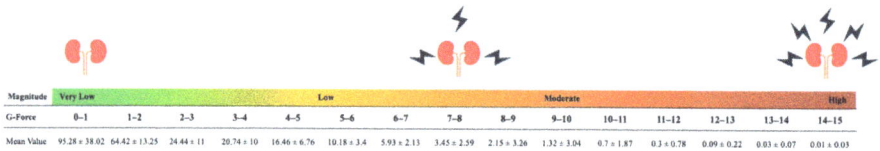

Figure 2. Mean values of impacts per minute associated with 15 g-force categories during off-road mountain running.

All sixteen impact-related variables were grouped in four different PC´s, explaining the 90.39% of total impacts cumulative variance. The 1st PC explained the 50.5% (EV = 8.08) of total variance, 2nd PC the 17.58% (EV = 2.81), 3rd PC the 13.05% (EV = 2.09), and 4th PC the 9.27% (EV = 1.48). Grouped variables and loadings are presented in Figure 3.

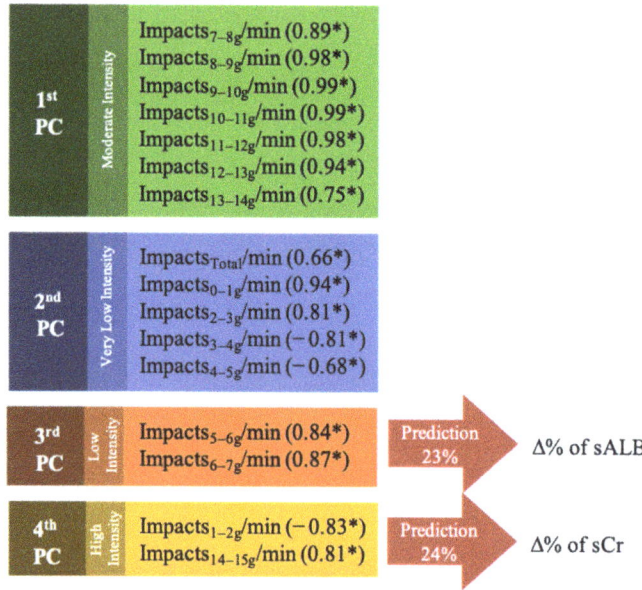

Figure 3. Principal component analysis extracted variables and loadings. * Loadings values.

In follow up to the abovementioned PCA results, those participants that met AKI diagnosis criteria (33.3% of participants) registered lower number of impacts in the 1–2 g category ($t = -2.42, p = 0.03$, $d = -1.45$, large effect size) but higher number of impacts in the 14–15 g category ($t = -3.1, p = 0.01$, $d = -1.58$, large effect size) (see Figure 4.). No differences we found in the 5–6 g or 6–7 g categories.

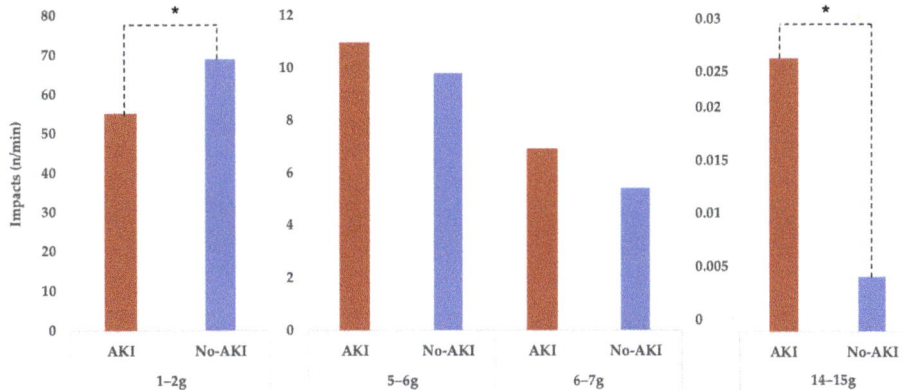

Figure 4. Differences between runners showing signs of AKI ($n = 6$) and those showing no signs of AKI ($n = 12$) regarding impacts per minute, grouped in four impact g-force categories. * The biggest difference between the AKI and no-AKI group is that the no-AKI group managed to run "smoother," keeping impacts in the lower impact load ranges, while avoiding higher impacts loads.

There were large statistical differences ($t = -6.24, p < 0.01, d = -1.47$, large effect size) between sCr pre-race (1.24 ± 0.28 mg/dL) and sCr post-race (1.74 ± 0.41 mg/dL), and large differences ($t = -2.78$, $p = 0.01, d = -1.47$, large effect size) in sALB pre-race (4.33 ± 1.29 IU/L) vs. post-race (5.01 ± 0.86 IU/L). The Δ% of sCr was predicted by the 4th PC in a 24% ($R^2 = 0.24, β = 44.03, p < 0.01$) and the Δ% of sALB by a 23% ($R^2 = 0.23, β = 100.55, p = 0.04$). Finally, USG as a hydration marker reported no differences between pre- and post-race measurements (1.01 ± 0.02 vs. 1.01 ± 0.01; $t = 1.02, p = 0.07$).

4. Discussion

Renal injury provoked by an indirect trauma has been reported in previous cases with no symptoms other than lumbar pain but with radiological findings such as subcapsular renal hematoma [14]. Some evidence suggests that urinary trauma could be present in non-contact sports such as off-road running [4,5,28]. It has been hypothesized that kidney mechanical trauma could mediate in the development of acute kidney injury after running [9]. This could be due to the kidneys' relative mobility during some actions as a downhill run at high speeds, change of directions, falls, and other high g-forces that could affect kidney movements and shaking. This relationship needs to be explored in future studies. The results of this study suggest that the 4th PC and 3rd PC of impact-related variables explained the Δ% of sCr and sALB between 23 to 24%. These findings indicate that the magnitude and number of impacts (g-forces) could have a potential role in the cumulative mechanical kidney trauma.

Despite kidneys being well protected by abdominal and back muscles, ribs, fat, renal pedicle, and ureteropelvic junction and supporting Gerota fascia in the retroperitoneum, they are also susceptible to internal movements [14,28]. Repeated sudden accelerations and decelerations may lead to renal contusions caused by the collision of kidneys in its surrounding tissues and structures like spine and ribs. These actions could lead to renal vasculatures affections, nephron damage, consequent hematuria, and other blood markers findings [29–31]. These accelerations and deceleration could be assessed using the variable impacts as proposed in this study. The impacts between 5–7 g explained the pre-post increase of sALB and the impacts of 1–2 g and 14–15 g explained the rise in sCr. Based on the literature [9], these results may suggest that both the volume and intensity of the impacts involved during renal contusions play a special role in acute kidney injury. It has been found that the Δ% of blood markers as serum creatine kinase and sCr could predict the external workload of wearable devices placed in L1–L3 by 40% and 27%, respectively [9]. This evidence supports the idea of a new hypothesis of mechanical kidney injury during endurance off-road running based on L1–L3 external workload data [9].

The results of the present study showed that MARG sensors could be used to register the impacts and g-forces that affect the lower back, which is the kidney´s nearest external structure of the body. MARG sensors could register vertical, anterior-posterior, and mediolateral forces using the integration of accelerometer, gyroscope, and magnetometer data. The g-forces provoked by sudden accelerations and decelerations may affect the kidneys. The number and magnitude of these impacts could be monitored using MARGs attached to the kidney´s nearest external structure of the body, the lower back. Kidneys typically extend from T12 to L3 and weigh 135–150 g, so the MARG positioning should be at this level despite a slight position change due to the kidney's free mobility resulting from both body positions and respiration [32].

The link between the sensors' external load and kidney trauma must be confirmed and discussed in future interventions. Previously, considering the cause of the increase in sCr may be indicative of kidney injury as well as massive muscle damage [33]. Although elevations in sCr in 33% of participants by itself should not be understood as kidney damage due to physical exercise, the rise in sALB could suggest transitory functional loss due to tubular or glomerular damage. In fact, there is evidence to suggest that proteins released into the bloodstream in high amounts (e.g., rhabdomyolysis) can overload kidney function, resulting in functional or subclinical damage reflected in an increase of sCr and sALB, respectively [34,35].

The cumulative small injuries during rough exercises as off-road mountain running might damage the kidney, resulting in AKI. Although there is no clear evidence that cumulative or subsequent AKI events contribute to future renal chronic conditions in athletes [1,36], there is enough evidence to suggest that athletes, coaches, and sports scientists should be concerned with controlling the kidney health of runners, monitoring those variables that can trigger AKI, and thus, preventing potential cases of this transitory kidney condition. Some preventive strategies have been proposed to endurance athletes such as optimal fluid and food intake, appropriate physical loading, rest, and acceptable recovery between efforts [3]. Monitoring physical load is essential and those external and internal variables that could affect not only kidney health but also general well-being should be assessed. Dehydration seems to be a factor that did not influence the AKI occurrence in this specific sample, as found in the results.

MARG units as wearable devices containing accelerometers, gyroscopes, and magnetometers allow trainers, athletes, and medical staff to monitor and control the physical external and internal loads involved during the off-road running. The information obtained would allow us to provide feedback on the kinematic behavior of the runner in an objective manner [37] and would facilitate the programming and prescription of training loads, preventing and mitigating the impact of AKI on the runner's health and performance.

These findings must be seen in light of some limitations. Considering that the cause of acute kidney injury is multifactorial, future studies may confirm the contribution of mechanical kidney damage in the increase of blood markers related to AKI. A global analysis of heat strain, metabolic responses, and dehydration should be made to explore the role of kidney mechanical trauma on AKI. The link of impacts assessed in the periphery of the body and mechanical trauma of hard connective tissues must be confirmed in future studies.

Also, it must be explored how much does prolonged massive g-forces impact runners during rough running (e.g., downhill, off-road, mountain) and produce kidney damage compared to similar heavy muscular exercise, but without the massive g-forces. Consequently, it should be explored if downhill running, sudden change of direction, falls, or other similar high magnitude actions produce greater damage than other running actions (e.g., uphill and flat running). Finally, there is a need to use other blood markers (e.g., Cystatin-C, NGAL, KIM-1) that allow researchers to differentiate AKI's and extreme muscular exercise's signs and symptoms. There is a need to review AKI's diagnosis criteria and its validity when applying it to sport sciences and medicine.

5. Conclusions

The results suggest that the magnitude and volume of running g-forces monitored with a MARG sensor attached to the lower back of off-road runners could predict the 24% change of serum creatinine and 23% change in serum albumin. These results must be confirmed in future research comparing similar heavy exercise with lower shock loads to the back and kidneys. Although these results may appear promising regarding the potential use of wearable devices to monitor cumulative mechanical kidney trauma in the future, greater understanding is required in the interaction of internal load (e.g., physiological responses) and external load (e.g., accelerations, impacts, decelerations) during prolonged exposure to vigorous repetitive exercise.

The results suggest that a decrease in the amount and magnitude of impacts throughout a session or between sessions can be a way to mitigate the possible collateral damage of acute kidney damage during off-road running. The foregoing considers, therefore, that the monitoring and control of training external and internal loads is essential for the prevention and recovery of AKI in off-road runners. In this sense, it is essential to provide constant feedback on running loads behavior and wearable MARG sensors could be used for these purposes.

Author Contributions: Conceptualization, D.R.-V.; methodology, D.R.-V., G.O., B.S.-U., and R.T.; software, D.R.-V., and J.P.-O.; validation, D.R.-V., G.O., B.S.-U., and R.T.; formal analysis, D.R.-V.; investigation, D.R.-V., B.S.-U., and J.P.-O.; resources, D.R.-V. and B.S.-U.; data curation, D.R.-V., J.P.-O., and I.M.-G.; writing—original draft preparation, D.R.-V., and I.M.-G.; writing—review and editing, D.R.-V., G.O., B.S.-U. and R.T.; supervision, D.R.-V., G.O., B.S.-U., and R.T.; project administration, D.R.-V., G.O., B.S.-U., and R.T.; funding acquisition, D.R.-V., G.O., B.S.-U., and R.T. All authors have read and agreed to the published version of the manuscript.

Funding: This research received no external funding.

Acknowledgments: Authors would like to express special thanks of gratitude to all participants and researchers of the CIDISAD and PROCESA laboratories for their administrative and technical support for the development of this study.

Conflicts of Interest: The authors declare no conflict of interest.

References

1. Hoffman, M.D.; Weiss, R.H. Does acute kidney injury from an ultramarathon increase the risk for greater subsequent injury? *Clin. J. Sport Med.* **2016**, *26*, 417–422. [CrossRef] [PubMed]
2. Beker, B.M.; Corleto, M.G.; Fieiras, C.; Musso, C.G. Novel acute kidney injury biomarkers: Their characteristics, utility and concerns. *Int. Urol. Nephrol.* **2018**, *50*, 705–713. [CrossRef] [PubMed]
3. Bongers, C.C.W.G.; Alsady, M.; Nijenhuis, T.; Tulp, A.D.M.; Eijsvogels, T.M.H.; Deen, P.M.T.; Hopman, M.T.E. Impact of acute versus prolonged exercise and dehydration on kidney function and injury. *Physiol. Rep.* **2018**, *6*. [CrossRef] [PubMed]
4. Urakami, S.; Ogawa, K.; Oka, S.; Hayashida, M.; Hagiwara, K.; Nagamoto, S.; Sakaguchi, K.; Yano, A.; Kurosawa, K.; Okaneya, T. Macroscopic hematuria caused by running-induced traumatic bladder mucosal contusions. *Iju. Case Rep.* **2019**, *2*, 27–29. [CrossRef]
5. Rojas-Valverde, D.; Olcina, G.; Sánchez-Ureña, B.; Pino-Ortega, J.; Martínez-Guardado, I.; Timón, R. Proteinuria and Bilirubinuria as Potential Risk Indicators of Acute Kidney Injury during Running in Outpatient Settings. *Medicina* **2020**, *56*, 562. [CrossRef] [PubMed]
6. Brophy, R.H.; Gamradt, S.C.; Barnes, R.P.; Powell, J.W.; DelPizzo, J.J.; Rodeo, S.A.; Warren, R.F. Kidney injuries in professional American football: Implications for management of an athlete with 1 functioning kidney. *Am. J. Sports Med.* **2008**, *36*, 85–90. [CrossRef] [PubMed]

7. Freeman, C.M.; Kelly, M.E.; Nason, G.J.; McGuire, B.B.; Kilcoyne, A.; Ryan, J.; Lennon, G.; Galvin, D.; Quinlan, D.; Mulvin, D. Renal Trauma: The Rugby Factor. *Curr. Urol.* **2015**, *8*, 133–137. [CrossRef]
8. Lipman, G.S.; Krabak, B.J.; Waite, B.L.; Logan, S.B.; Menon, A.; Chan, G.K. A Prospective Cohort Study of Acute Kidney Injury in Multi-stage Ultramarathon Runners: The Biochemistry in Endurance Runner Study (BIERS). *Res. Sports Med.* **2014**, *22*, 185–192. [CrossRef]
9. Rojas-Valverde, D.; Sánchez-Ureña, B.; Pino-Ortega, J.; Gómez-Carmona, C.; Gutiérrez-Vargas, R.; Timón, R.; Olcina, G. External Workload Indicators of Muscle and Kidney Mechanical Injury in Endurance Trail Running. *Int. J. Environ. Res. Public Health* **2019**, *16*, 3909. [CrossRef]
10. Gutiérrez-Vargas, R.; Martín-Rodríguez, S.; Sánchez-Ureña, B.; Rodríguez-Montero, A.; Salas-Cabrera, J.; Gutiérrez-Vargas, J.C.; Simunic, B.; Rojas-Valverde, D. Biochemical and Muscle Mechanical Postmarathon Changes in Hot and Humid Conditions. *J. Strength Cond. Res.* **2020**, *34*, 847–856. [CrossRef]
11. Rojas-Valverde, D.; Olcina, G.; Gutiérrez-Vargas, R.; Crowe, J. Heat Strain, External Workload, and Chronic Kidney Disease in Tropical Settings: Are Endurance Athletes Exposed? *Front. Physiol.* **2019**, *10*, 1403. [CrossRef] [PubMed]
12. Kao, W.-F.; Hou, S.-K.; Chiu, Y.-H.; Chou, S.-L.; Kuo, F.-C.; Wang, S.-H.; Chen, J.-J. Effects of 100-km Ultramarathon on Acute Kidney Injury. *Clin. J. Sport Med.* **2015**, *25*, 49–54. [CrossRef] [PubMed]
13. Junglee, N.A.; Di Felice, U.; Dolci, A.; Fortes, M.B.; Jibani, M.M.; Lemmey, A.B.; Walsh, N.P.; Macdonald, J.H. Exercising in a hot environment with muscle damage: Effects on acute kidney injury biomarkers and kidney function. *Am. J. Physiol. Ren. Physiol.* **2013**, *305*, F813–F820. [CrossRef] [PubMed]
14. Kasikcioglu, E.; Kayserilioglu, A.; Kadioglu, A. Can Renal Hematoma Occur without a Direct Trauma During Exercise? A Case Report. *J. Sports Sci. Med.* **2004**, *3*, 101–103. [PubMed]
15. Rojas-Valverde, D.; Gómez-Carmona, C.D.; Gutiérrez-Vargas, R.; Pino-Ortega, J. From big data mining to technical sport reports: The case of inertial measurement units. *Bmj Open Sport Exerc. Med.* **2019**, *5*, e000565. [CrossRef]
16. Lynn, R.; Pfitzer, R.; Rogers, R.R.; Ballmann, C.G.; Williams, T.D.; Marshall, M.R. Step-Counting Validity of Wrist-Worn Activity Monitors During Activities with Fixed Upper Extremities. *J. Meas. Phys. Behav.* **2020**, *1*, 1–7. [CrossRef]
17. Rojas-Valverde, D.; Ramírez, J.A.U.; Sánchez-Ureña, B.; Gutiérrez-Vargas, R. Influence of Altitude and Environmental Temperature on Muscle Functional and Mechanical Activation After 30' Time Trial Run. *Mhsalud Rev. Cienc. Mov. Hum. Y Salud.* **2020**, *17*, 1–15. [CrossRef]
18. Toth, L.P.; Park, S.; Pittman, W.L.; Sarisaltik, D.; Hibbing, P.R.; Morton, A.L.; Springer, C.M.; Crouter, S.E.; Bassett, D.R. Effects of Brief Intermittent Walking Bouts on Step Count Accuracy of Wearable Devices. *J. Meas. Phys. Behav.* **2019**, *2*, 13–21. [CrossRef]
19. Rico-González, M.; Los Arcos, A.; Rojas-Valverde, D.; Clemente, F.M.; Pino-Ortega, J. A Survey to Assess the Quality of the Data Obtained by Radio-Frequency Technologies and Microelectromechanical Systems to Measure External Workload and Collective Behavior Variables in Team Sports. *Sensors* **2020**, *20*, 2271. [CrossRef]
20. Oliva-Lozano, J.M.; Martín-Fuentes, I.; Muyor, J.M. Validity and Reliability of an Inertial Device for Measuring Dynamic Weight-Bearing Ankle Dorsiflexion. *Sensors* **2020**, *20*, 399. [CrossRef]
21. Gómez-Carmona, C.D.; Bastida-Castillo, A.; González-Custodio, A.; Olcina, G.; Pino-Ortega, J. Using an Inertial Device (WIMU PRO^{TM}) to Quantify Neuromuscular Load in Running. Reliability, Convergent Validity and Influence of Type of Surface and Device Location. *J. Strength Cond. Res.* **2019**, *34*, 365–373, Epub: Ahead of print.
22. Gómez-Carmona, C.D.; Bastida-Castillo, A.; García-Rubio, J.; Ibáñez, S.J.; Pino-Ortega, J. Static and dynamic reliability of WIMU PRO^{TM} accelerometers according to anatomical placement. *Proc. Inst. Mech. Eng. Part P J. Sports Eng. Technol.* **2018**, *233*, 238–248, Epub: Ahead of print.
23. Lopes, J.A.; Jorge, S. The RIFLE and AKIN classifications for acute kidney injury: A critical and comprehensive review. *Clin. Kidney J.* **2013**, *6*, 8–14. [CrossRef] [PubMed]
24. Wyness, S.P.; Hunsaker, J.J.H.; Snow, T.M.; Genzen, J.R. Evaluation and analytical validation of a handheld digital refractometer for urine specific gravity measurement. *Pract. Lab. Med.* **2016**, *5*, 65–74. [CrossRef]
25. Casa, D.J.; Armstrong, L.E.; Hillman, S.K.; Montain, S.J.; Reiff, R.V.; Rich, B.S.E.; Roberts, W.O.; Stone, J.A. National Athletic Trainers' Association Position Statement: Fluid Replacement for Athletes. *J. Athl. Train.* **2000**, *35*, 212–224.

26. Oliva-Lozano, J.M.; Rojas-Valverde, D.; Gómez-Carmona, C.D.; Fortes, V.; Pino-Ortega, J. Impact of Contextual Variables On The Representative External Load Profile Of Spanish Professional Soccer Match-Play: A Full Season Study. *Eur. J. Sport Sci.* **2020**, 1–22. [CrossRef]
27. Rojas-Valverde, D.; Pino-Ortega, J.; Gómez-Carmona, C.D.; Rico-González, M. A Systematic Review of Methods and Criteria Standard Proposal for the Use of Principal Component Analysis in Team's Sports Science. *Int. J. Environ. Res. Public Health* **2020**, *17*, 8712. [CrossRef]
28. Holmes, F.C.; Hunt, J.J.; Sevier, T.L. Renal injury in sport. *Curr. Sports Med. Rep.* **2003**, *2*, 103–109. [CrossRef]
29. Abarbanel, J.; Benet, A.E.; Lask, D.; Kimche, D. Sports Hematuria. *J. Urol.* **1990**, *143*, 887–890. [CrossRef]
30. Erlich, T.; Kitrey, N.D. Renal trauma: The current best practice. *Adv. Urol.* **2018**, *10*, 295–303. [CrossRef]
31. Schmidlin, F.; Farshad, M.; Bidaut, L.; Barbezat, M.; Becker, C.; Niederer, P.; Graber, P. Biomechanical analysis and clinical treatment of blunt renal trauma. *Swiss Surg.* **1998**, 237–243.
32. Chiva, L.M.; Magrina, J. Chapter 2—Abdominal and Pelvic Anatomy. In *Principles of Gynecologic Oncology Surgery*; Ramirez, P.T., Frumovitz, M., Abu-Rustum, N.R., Eds.; Elsevier: Amsterdam, The Netherlands, 2018; pp. 3–49. ISBN 978-0-323-42878-1.
33. Samra, M.; Abcar, A.C. False Estimates of Elevated Creatinine. *Perm. J.* **2012**, *16*, 51. [CrossRef] [PubMed]
34. Gameiro, J.; Agapito Fonseca, J.; Jorge, S.; Lopes, J.A. Acute Kidney Injury Definition and Diagnosis: A Narrative Review. *J. Clin. Med.* **2018**, *7*, 307. [CrossRef] [PubMed]
35. Ronco, C.; Kellum, J.A.; Haase, M. Subclinical AKI is still AKI. *Crit. Care* **2012**, *16*, 313. [CrossRef] [PubMed]
36. Rojas-Valverde, D.; Sánchez-Ureña, B.; Crowe, J.; Timón, R.; Olcina, G.J. Exertional Rhabdomyolysis and Acute Kidney Injury in Endurance Sports: A Systematic Review. *Eur. J. Sport Sci.* **2020**, 1–28. [CrossRef]
37. Wieringa, F.P.; Broers, N.J.H.; Kooman, J.P.; Van Der Sande, F.M.; Van Hoof, C. Wearable sensors: Can they benefit patients with chronic kidney disease? *Expert Rev. Med. Devices* **2017**, *14*, 505–519. [CrossRef]

Publisher's Note: MDPI stays neutral with regard to jurisdictional claims in published maps and institutional affiliations.

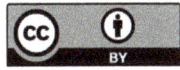

© 2020 by the authors. Licensee MDPI, Basel, Switzerland. This article is an open access article distributed under the terms and conditions of the Creative Commons Attribution (CC BY) license (http://creativecommons.org/licenses/by/4.0/).

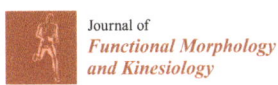

Journal of
Functional Morphology and Kinesiology

Article

Effect of Video Observation and Motor Imagery on Simple Reaction Time in Cadet Pilots

Felice Sirico [1,*], Veronica Romano [1], Anna Maria Sacco [1], Immacolata Belviso [1], Vittoria Didonna [2], Daria Nurzynska [1], Clotilde Castaldo [1], Stefano Palermi [1], Giuseppe Sannino [1], Elisabetta Della Valle [1], Stefania Montagnani [1] and Franca Di Meglio [1]

1 Department of Public Health, University of Naples "Federico II", 80131 Naples, Italy; veronica.romano@unina.it (V.R.); annamaria.sacco@unina.it (A.M.S.); immacolata.belviso@unina.it (I.B.); dariaanna.nurzynska@unina.it (D.N.); clotilde.castaldo@unina.it (C.C.); stefanopalermi8@gmail.com (S.P.); giuseppe.sannino88@gmail.com (G.S.); elisabetta.dellavalle@unina.it (E.D.V.); montagna@unina.it (S.M.); franca.dimeglio@unina.it (F.D.M.)
2 Italian Air Force Academy, 80078 Pozzuoli, Italy; viria92did@gmail.com
* Correspondence: felice.sirico2@unina.it

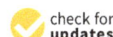

Received: 10 October 2020; Accepted: 3 December 2020; Published: 5 December 2020

Abstract: Neuromotor training can improve motor performance in athletes and patients. However, few data are available about their effect on reaction time (RT). We investigated the influence of video observation/motor imagery (VO/MI) on simple RT to visual and auditory stimuli. The experimental group comprised 21 cadets who performed VO/MI training over 4 weeks. Nineteen cadets completed a sham intervention as control. The main outcome measure was RT to auditory and visual stimuli for the upper and lower limbs. The RT to auditory stimuli improved significantly post-intervention in both groups (control vs. experimental mean change for upper limbs: −40 ms vs. −40 ms, $p = 0.0008$; for lower limbs: −50 ms vs. −30 ms, $p = 0.0174$). A trend towards reduced RT to visual stimuli was observed (for upper limbs: −30 ms vs. −20 ms, $p = 0.0876$; for lower limbs: −30 ms vs. −20 ms, $p = 0.0675$). The interaction term was not significant. Only the specific VO/MI training produced a linear correlation between the improvement in the RT to auditory and visual stimuli for the upper ($r = 0.703$) and lower limbs ($r = 0.473$). In conclusion, VO/MI training does not improve RT when compared to control, but it may be useful in individuals who need to simultaneously develop a fast response to different types of stimuli.

Keywords: reaction time; pilots; motor imagery; video observation

1. Introduction

The time to respond to an external stimulus (reaction time) is the time lapse between the presentation of a stimulus and the onset of a voluntary response in a subject. The reaction time can be defined as the interval required to perceive the stimulus, process the information, fulfill an appropriate decision-making process, and initiate a motor task as a response [1]. Such a sequence of events adding to the reaction time is typical of real-life tasks and plays a critical role in many human activities related to sport or the professional performance of drivers, military personnel, security guards, or pilots. In neurophysiology, reaction time represents a valid indicator of an individual's sensorimotor coordination and performance [2]. Three different types of reaction time can be described, based on the relationship between stimulus and response: simple, recognition, and choice reaction time [3]. In simple reaction time studies, there is one stimulus (auditory, visual or tactile) and one response. In recognition reaction time studies, stimuli to be responded to are interspersed with distracters that should not be followed with a response. In choice reaction time studies, several stimuli require different responses.

Reduction of reaction time is a desirable aim of intervention, both in the general population and its subsets, including athletes (e.g., swimmers or sprinters starting off the block in response to auditory stimulus or volleyball players pushing off in response to visual stimulus), patients affected by diabetes or osteoporosis (e.g., for fall prevention) [4], youths with intellectual disabilities, and patients with acoustic or visual impairment [5,6].

The reaction times of aviation pilots to auditory or visual stimuli and the skills in the execution of complex movements in response to these stimuli are of paramount importance during flight [7]. Aviation requires a combination of decision-making and kinesthetic skills. Many tasks during aircraft flying require continuous visual and auditory monitoring of the cues outside and inside the aircraft. Hence, the basic requirements of the pilot profession include fast and efficient information processing and fast and accurate reaction time [8]. Kennedy et al. [9] found that greater intra-individual variability in reaction time had an adverse impact on the ability of the pilot to maintain control of the aircraft in a flight simulator. These observations highlight the importance of the reduction of reaction time to different types of stimuli for the multitude of different tasks.

The motor imagery (MI) technique, trying to develop precise mental representations of the motor ability, led to improved performance of skilled movements [10]. Similarly, the video observation (VO) aids short-term motor skills learning [11]. These results can have the mirror neurons system as neurofunctional and neuroanatomical basis, a system able to facilitate subsequent movement executions by directly matching the observed action to the internal simulation of that action [12].

While it is known that MI and VO can exert positive effects on motor skill performance [13], few data are available regarding the effectiveness of these neuromotor training techniques in the reduction of the reaction times. Therefore, the aim of the present study was to investigate the influence of MI and VO on the simple reaction time to auditory and visual stimuli.

2. Materials and Methods

2.1. Subjects

The study protocol was approved in advance by the Ethical Committee of the University of Naples Federico II (22 March 2017, protocol number 58/17). Each subject provided written informed consent before participating. Participants were recruited on a voluntary basis among adult (age >18 years) male pilot cadets enrolled at the Italian Air Force Academy in Pozzuoli (Italy). Subjects with painful conditions during the three previous months and subjects affected by known orthopedic, rheumatologic, visual, acoustic, or neurological diseases that could interfere with the correct execution of the study protocol were excluded.

2.2. Procedure

Before randomization, all eligible subjects performed a pre-test evaluation of the imagery ability, using the revised movement imagery questionnaire (MIQ-R) [14]. The MIQ-R scores were collected at baseline and compared between groups to test for the homogeneity in imagery ability but were not considered in randomization or as an outcome measure.

The auditory and visual reaction times were measured using the Optojump device (Microgate, Bolzano, Italy), a previously validated and used tool for the measurement of reaction times [5,15–17]. This device is based on an infrared led technology and composed of transmitting and receiving parallel bars. To measure the reaction time for the lower limbs, the bars were positioned on the floor and the subject stood between the bars. The subject received the instruction to jump, lifting both feet off the floor, in response to an auditory (sound produced by the device) or a visual (appearance of a green ball on the device screen) stimulus. For the measurement of the upper-limb reaction time, the bars were positioned on a table with adjustable height. The subject stood in front of the table and the device height was set to allow positioning of both palms flat on the table between bars with full bilateral elbow extension and wrist extension. The subject received the instruction to lift both hands in response to auditory or visual stimulus. Each subject was allowed a single practice attempt to gain confidence with the equipment. All tests were supervised by a trained physician who was blinded to the group allocation.

The main outcome measure was the reaction time expressed in milliseconds (ms). Auditory and visual reaction times for lower and upper limbs were assessed during the same session, in the following order: three trials of auditory reaction time for lower limbs, three trials of visual reaction time for lower limbs, three trials of auditory reaction time for upper limbs, and three trials of visual reaction time for upper limbs. The mean value of each triplicate measurement was calculated for statistical analysis.

Subjects were randomly assigned to the control or experimental group, using dedicated online software (https://www.sealedenvelope.com/simple-randomiser/v1/lists). Following randomization, each subject received an identical-looking USB pen drive containing a video demonstrating the motor tasks necessary to complete either sham (control group) or specific (experimental group) VO/MI intervention protocol. All cadets participated in a training session dedicated to the principles and aim of the VO and MI techniques. Subjects were informed not to discuss the protocols, observe others during VO/MI protocol execution, or share any information about the study throughout its duration.

The VO/MI intervention comprised individual, supervised and non-directed sessions, carried out regularly for 4 weeks. For both sham VO/MI (control) and specific VO/MI (experimental) groups, each task represented in the video was repeated three times in a loop. No instructions were provided in the video about the observed tasks and their subsequent imaging and execution. The video, watched on a laptop 9.7" screen, had no audio, except for the sound in the task related to the auditory stimulation reaction time assessment observed by the specific VO/MI group.

Each VO session was followed by an MI session and then the actual movement execution. All subjects were instructed to keep their eyes closed during MI. The whole routine, involving imagining the tasks observed in the video and actual movements, was performed by the cadets, always using the same equipment and at the same time of the day. Recorded tasks were performed by a male age-matched model wearing the leisure uniforms worn by all cadets at the Academy. Subjects allocated to the experimental group watched a video depicting the auditory and visual reaction time assessment, which was identical to that carried out during the baseline and end-point assessments. Hence, the experimental group performed an MI activity and then the actual movements based on VO aimed at improvement of auditory and visual reaction times. Subjects in the control group watched a video depicting activity included in an everyday physical training program (running, static bench, full push-up, standing toe touch), performed in the gym, followed by VO and MI procedures involving those activities. Thus, the VO/MI practiced by the control group was not related in any way to the end task for which the reaction time was measured.

2.3. Statistical Analysis

The main outcome of the study was to assess the change in the reaction time to auditory and visual stimulation following a neuromotor intervention comprising specific VO/MI compared with a sham neuromotor intervention. Therefore, the null hypothesis of the study was that the specific VO/MI would have no impact on the reaction times.

The distribution of continuous variables was assessed using the Shapiro–Wilk test and reported as mean ± SD. The MIQ-R scores were considered ordinal and reported as median and interquartile range (IQR) for visual and kinesthetic subscales. Data were analyzed by a Mixed Model ANOVA. Time was considered as within-subjects factor (baseline and post-intervention evaluation). Sham and specific interventions (group variable) were considered as the between-subjects factor. Interaction between time and group was investigated. The correlation between the Δ Reaction Time to auditory and the Δ Reaction Time to visual stimulus was assessed by Pearson correlation coefficients. All tests were considered significant if the p value was less than 0.05. Data analysis was performed using STATA software (StataCorp. v.12, College Station, TX, USA).

3. Results

In total, 41 males were assessed for eligibility. One cadet was excluded due to a recent orthopedic injury. Included subjects were randomly assigned to the control ($n = 19$) or intervention ($n = 21$) group. The mean age was 21.05 years (SD 0.97, range 20–23) in the control group and 20.7 years (SD 0.96, range 20–23) in the experimental group ($p = 0.573$). The MIQ-R scores were similar between groups (control group: median 20, IQR 19–21; experimental group: median 19, IQR 18–20, $p = 0.105$ for the kinesthetic subscale and control: median 19, IQR 18–19; experimental: median 17, IQR 17–19, $p = 0.101$ for the visual subscale).

The mean scores for the reaction time to auditory and visual stimuli for the upper and lower limbs pre- and post-intervention are reported in Figure 1 and the results of the analysis are reported in Table 1. The reaction time to auditory stimuli for the upper and lower limbs post-intervention improved significantly in both groups (control: mean change −40 ms, SD 40, experimental: mean change −40 ms, SD 80 for upper limbs; control: mean change −50 ms, SD 140, experimental: mean change −30 ms, SD 70 for lower limbs). A trend towards reduced reaction time to visual stimuli for upper and lower limbs was also observed in both groups (control: mean change −30 ms, SD 90, experimental: mean change −20 ms, SD 100 for upper limbs; control: mean change −30 ms, SD 90, experimental: mean change −20 ms, SD 80 for lower limbs). The effect of time was significant in all groups. The group effect for auditory and visual RT was not significant in upper limbs, while it was significant in lower limbs. In all comparisons, interaction term was not significant.

While results showed similar improvement in the reaction times in both groups, the correlation between the reduction of the reaction times to visual and auditory stimuli differed between the groups (Figure 2). In the experimental group, reductions in the reaction times to visual and auditory stimuli were significantly correlated, with a high coefficient, for both upper ($r = 0.703$) and lower limbs ($r = 0.473$). Conversely, this correlation was not significant in the control group ($r = 0.262$ for the upper and $r = 0.09$ for the lower limbs).

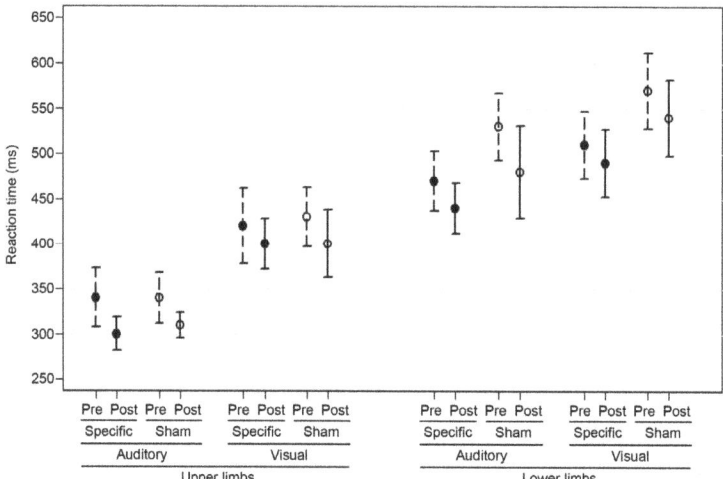

Figure 1. Reaction times to visual and auditory stimuli for upper and lower limbs in the experimental (specific VO/MI) and control (sham VO/MI) groups. Data are reported in milliseconds as a mean and 95% confidence interval. Solid circle indicates experimental group (specific intervention), hollow circle indicates control group (sham intervention).

Table 1. Reaction times (RT) to auditory and visual stimuli for the upper and lower limbs pre- and post- VO/MI training in the control and experimental groups.

Limbs RT in ms	Control Group			Experimental Group		
	Pre, Mean (SD)	Post, Mean (SD)	Change, Mean (SD)	Pre, Mean (SD)	Post, Mean (SD)	Change, Mean (SD)
Auditory, upper	340 (60)	310 (30)	−40 (40)	340 (70)	300 (40)	−40 (80)
Visual, upper	430 (70)	400 (80)	−30 (90)	420 (90)	400 (60)	−20 (100)
Auditory, lower	530 (80)	480 (110)	−50 (140)	470 (70)	440 (60)	−30 (70)
Visual, lower	570 (90)	540 (90)	−30 (90)	510 (80)	490 (80)	−20 (80)

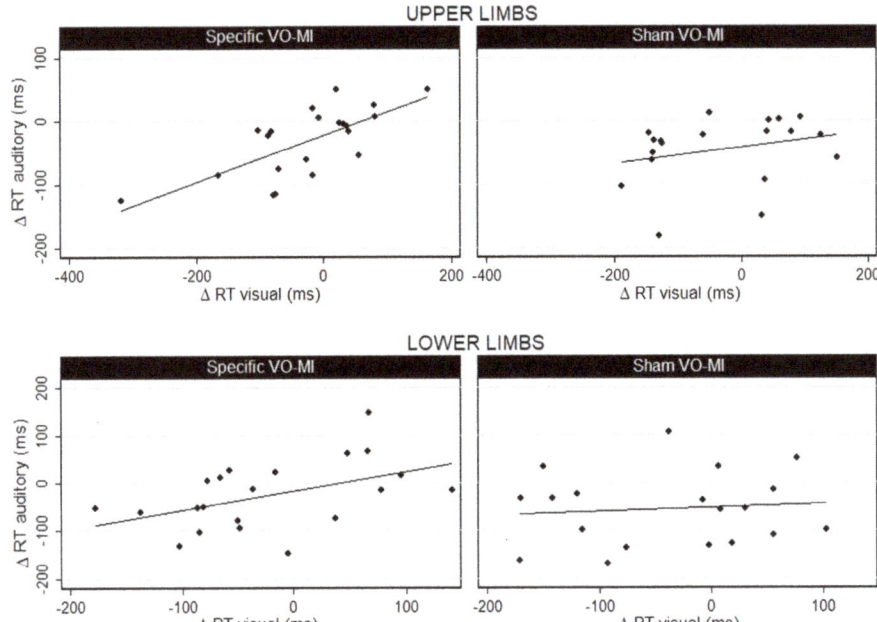

Figure 2. Correlation between the reduction in the reaction time (ΔRT) to visual and auditory stimuli for upper and lower limbs in the experimental (specific VO/MI) and control (sham VO/MI) groups.

4. Discussion

Our study demonstrated that a neuromotor intervention comprising a specific VO/MI did not significantly improve reaction times to visual and auditory stimuli for upper or lower limbs when compared with controls. However, the correlation between the reduction in reaction time to visual and auditory stimuli was demonstrated only in the experimental group. Importantly, we observed that the reaction times for upper and lower limbs to auditory stimuli in both groups were lower than those registered for visual stimuli at baseline. Following the specific or sham VO/MI training, reductions in reaction times in the experimental and control groups were always more significant for the auditory than visual stimuli.

Specific MI/VO sessions were programmed to respect the elements of successful interventions identified by Schuster et al. [18]; these were individual, supervised and non-directed sessions, added after physical practice. Furthermore, the whole specific routine (VO followed by MI followed by movement execution) was based on the approach suggested by Holmes and Collins [19], which incorporates physical, environment, timing, task, learning, emotion, and perspective (PETTLEP) elements into imagery. Monitoring and adjusting for as many PETTLEP elements as feasible were recently proposed to optimize the intervention outcome and to maximize the functional equivalence of imaged and actual task execution, since the PETTLEP technique was associated with a greater ease and/or vividness of the MI [20]. Its effectiveness was observed in several fields where the best possible performance of movement is crucial, such as sport, surgery or music [21]. Despite those previously reported positive effects in the performance of the movements, in our study, the VO/MI technique incorporating PETTLEP elements showed no advantage in improving reaction times to auditory and visual stimuli over the control group, in which those principles were not respected. This is in contrast with findings published by Simons et al. [22], who found that brain-training interventions improve performance in the trained tasks but not in the unrelated tasks. Nevertheless, their literature review did not include studies of MI or VO but focused on studies aimed at improving cognitive skills rather than simple reaction times.

Knowing that the reaction times positively correlate with physical fitness level [23], it can be argued that mandatory participation in the physical training program, that is included in the schedule of all Air Force Academy students, could have contributed to the improved reaction times observed in both control and intervention groups. Indeed, it was observed that students who exercised regularly had shorter reaction times than those who lead a sedentary life [24]. Shorter simple reaction times were also observed in elderly diabetic patients with or without neuropathy after moderate or intense supervised exercise program compared with pre-training [25]. Similarly, reaction time improved in children and adolescents with mild intellectual disability who participated in physical fitness training programs, compared to a control group [26]. Recent studies suggest that the negative effects of stressful conditions on workplace performance and, presumably, reaction time could be overcome by physical training [27,28].

The reaction time represents a complex neuromotor skill and it can be influenced by several external and internal factors, including type of stimulus (auditory, visual, or tactile), sex, age, physical fitness, level of fatigue, distraction, alcohol, personality type, dominant limb, biological rhythm, and health [13,23,29,30]. Accordingly, the study population selected for our study was homogeneous by gender, age, instruction level, biological rhythm, professional demands, instruction, and physical fitness, owing to a common resident training program applied to the entire sample by the Air Force Academy. Although it was not possible to control for all variables able to influence reaction times, many of the considered factors were homogeneously distributed in the study population.

Admittedly, the present study has still some limitations related to the subject of the investigation. Because studies of VO/MI effects on reaction time are lacking, we calculated the sample size for our study based on similar data on motor performance published elsewhere [13] and assumed a reduction of 150 ms in the auditory and visual reaction time as clinically significant. The absence of significant differences between groups could be caused by a high type II error with a low power of the results, due to the limited sample. As stated above, our study sample is represented by a highly homogenous population of the same gender, age, social status, lifestyle, education and physical activity. While this consideration allowed us to achieve an internal validity of the study design and results, at the same time, it may limit the generalization of the results. Regarding the choice of intervention, recent data suggested that a combination of model observation and self-observation had better short-term effects on motor performance than each VO method applied separately [11]. Nevertheless, only ideal model observation was used in the present study to explore, for the first time, its effect on the simple reaction time in association with MI. Further studies may be required to evaluate if the combination of both VO variants is more beneficial. Additional uncontrolled factors influencing the results of our study are placebo and expectation effects. Our choice of sham intervention in the control group, in which the VO/MI procedure was followed, but it was not related to the end task for which the reaction time was measured, allowed us to create an active control group. Recent studies indicate, however, that it may not be sufficient for eliminating a placebo effect, since the experimental and active control group can develop different expectations of improvement, even if interventions are incomparable [31].

In activities that take place in relatively unpredictable and constantly changing environment, movements have to be continuously adapted. Thus, developing physical and motor capabilities is as important as improving sensory and cognitive skills. This is particularly relevant for, but not limited to, open-skill sport activities [32]. In closed-skill sports (swimming, running), reaction time to auditory stimulus is often determinant for success. Additionally, in some professional activities, such as aviation, reaction must follow prompts of different types, including visual and auditory stimuli. The current study found that specific VO/MI training related to the end task, whereby the reaction time is measured, allows a parallel reduction in the reaction time for both types of stimuli. Further research in the cognitive and neurophysiological field, possibly incorporating the concept of spatiotemporal window for multisensory integration [33], is needed to explore how this correlation influences the information process; this could lead not only to better simple reaction time, but also to better recognition or choice reaction times.

5. Conclusions

In conclusion, we observed that the reaction times for upper and lower limbs to auditory stimuli were always lower, at baseline, than those registered for visual stimuli. The neuromotor training comprising specific VO and MI procedures in the experimental group did not determine a significantly higher reduction in the simple reaction time to auditory and visual stimuli than the sham procedure in the control group. Indeed, a significant reduction of reaction time to auditory stimulus and a trend towards reduction of reaction time to visual stimulus was observed post-intervention for the upper and lower limbs in both groups. Only the specific VO/MI training, however, produced a linear correlation between the improvement in the reaction time to auditory and visual stimuli. Interestingly, the reductions in reaction times in the experimental and control groups were always more significant for the auditory than visual stimuli. These findings could be crucial in training programs for aviation cadets and other professionals who need to improve their reaction times to a multitude of stimuli.

Author Contributions: Conceptualization, F.S., V.R. and G.S.; Data curation, I.B. and V.D.; Formal analysis, A.M.S. and C.C.; Investigation, A.M.S., I.B. and D.N.; Methodology, F.S. and E.D.V.; Project administration, S.M. and F.D.M.; Resources, V.D. and G.S.; Supervision, F.S.; Validation, E.D.V. and F.D.M.; Visualization, C.C. and S.P.; Writing—Original draft, A.M.S., S.P. and F.D.M.; Writing—Review & editing, V.R., D.N. and S.M. All authors have read and agreed to the published version of the manuscript.

Funding: This research received no external funding.

Conflicts of Interest: The authors declare no conflict of interest.

References

1. Taimela, S. Factors affecting reaction-time testing and the interpretation of results. *Percept. Mot. Ski.* **1991**, *73* (Suppl. 3), 1195–1202.
2. Balakrishnan, G.; Uppinakudru, G.; Girwar, S.G.; Bangera, S.; Raghavendra, D.A.; Thangavel, D. A comparative study on visual choice reaction time for different colors in females. *Neur. Res. Int.* **2014**, *2014*, 301473.
3. Miller, J.O.; Low, K. Motor processes in simple, go/no-go, and choice reaction time tasks: A psychophysiological analysis. *J. Exp. Psychol Hum. Percept. Perform.* **2001**, *27*, 266–289.
4. Palermi, S.; Sacco, A.M.; Belviso, I.; Marino, N.; Gambardella, F.; Loiaco, C.; Sirico, F. Effectiveness of Tai Chi on Balance Improvement in Type 2 Diabetes Patients: A Systematic Review and Meta-Analysis. *J. Aging Phys. Act.* **2020**, *3*, 1–11.
5. Spera, R.; Belviso, I.; Sirico, F.; Palermi, S.; Massa, B.; Mazzeo, F.; Montesano, P. Jump and balance test in judo athletes with or without visual impairments. *J. Hum. Sport Exerc.* **2019**, *14*, S937–S947.
6. Metter, E.J.; Schrager, M.; Ferrucci, L.; Talbot, L.A. Evaluation of movement speed and reaction time as predictors of all-cause mortality in men. *J. Gerontol. A Biol. Sci. Med. Sci.* **2005**, *60*, 840–846. [PubMed]

7. Bennett, S.A. Pilot workload and fatigue on four intra-European routes: A 12-month mixed-methods evaluation. *J. Risk Res.* **2019**, *22*, 983–1003.
8. Barkhuizen, W.; Schepers, J.; Coetzee, J. Rate of information processing and reaction time of aircraft pilots and non-pilots. *SA J. Ind. Psychol.* **2002**, *28*, 67–76.
9. Kennedy, Q.; Taylor, J.; Heraldez, D.; Noda, A.; Lazzeroni, L.C.; Yesavage, J. Intraindividual variability in basic reaction time predicts middle-aged and older pilots' flight simulator performance. *J. Gerontol. B Psychol. Sci. Soc. Sci.* **2013**, *68*, 487–494.
10. Fontani, G.; Migliorini, S.; Benocci, R.; Facchini, A.; Casini, M.; Corradeschi, F. Effect of mental imagery on the development of skilled motor actions. *Percept. Mot. Ski.* **2007**, *105*, 803–826.
11. Nishizawa, H.; Kimura, T. Enhancement of motor skill learning by a combination of ideal model-observation and self-observation. *J. Phys. Ther. Sci.* **2017**, *29*, 1555–1560. [PubMed]
12. Sale, P.; Franceschini, M. Action observation and mirror neuron network: A tool for motor stroke rehabilitation. *Eur. J. Phys. Rehabil. Med.* **2012**, *48*, 313–318. [PubMed]
13. Battaglia, C.; D'Artibale, E.; Fiorilli, G.; Piazza, M.; Tsopani, D.; Giombini, A.; Calcagno, G.; di Cagno, A. Use of video observation and motor imagery on jumping performance in national rhythmic gymnastics athletes. *Hum. Mov. Sci.* **2014**, *38*, 225–234.
14. Hall, C.R.; Martin, K.A. Measuring movement imagery abilities: A revision of the Movement Imagery Questionnaire. *J. Ment. Imag.* **1997**, *21*, 143–154.
15. Bosquet, L.; Berryman, N.; Dupuy, O. A comparison of 2 optical timing systems designed to measure flight time and contact time during jumping and hopping. *J. Strength Cond. Res.* **2009**, *23*, 2660–2665. [PubMed]
16. Di Cagno, A.; Baldari, C.; Battaglia, C.; Monteiro, M.D.; Pappalardo, A.; Piazza, M.; Guidetti, L. Factors influencing performance of competitive and amateur rhythmic gymnastics-gender differences. *J. Sci. Med. Sport* **2009**, *12*, 411–416.
17. Mroczek, D.; Kawczyński, A.; Chmura, J. Changes of reaction time and blood lactate concentration of elite volleyball players during a game. *J. Hum. Kinet.* **2011**, *28*, 73–78.
18. Schuster, C.; Hilfiker, R.; Amft, O.; Scheidhauer, A.; Andrews, B.; Butler, J.; Ettlin, K.; Ettlin, T. Best practice for motor imagery: A systematic literature review on motor imagery training elements in five different disciplines. *BMC Med.* **2011**, *9*, 75.
19. Holmes, P.S.; Collins, D.J. The PETTLEP approach to motor imagery: A functional equivalence model for sport psychologists. *J. Appl. Sport Psychol.* **2001**, *13*, 60–83.
20. Anuar, N.; Williams, S.E.; Cumming, J. Do the physical and environment PETTLEP elements predict sport imagery ability? *Eur. J. Sport Sci.* **2017**, *17*, 1319–1327.
21. Collins, D.; Carson, H.J. The future for PETTLEP: A modern perspective on an effective and established tool. *Curr. Opin. Psychol.* **2017**, *16*, 12–16. [CrossRef] [PubMed]
22. Simons, D.J.; Boot, W.R.; Charness, N.; Gathercole, S.E.; Chabris, C.F.; Hambrick, D.Z.; Stine, M.L.A.E. Do "brain-training" programs work? *Psychol. Sci. Public Interest* **2016**, *17*, 103–186. [CrossRef] [PubMed]
23. Brisswalter, J.; Arcelin, R.; Audiffren, M.; Delignières, D. Influence of physical exercise on simple reaction time: Effect of physical fitness. *Percept. Mot. Ski.* **1997**, *85*, 1019–1027. [CrossRef] [PubMed]
24. Jain, A.; Bansal, R.; Kumar, A.; Singh, K.D. A comparative study of visual and auditory reaction times on the basis of gender and physical activity levels of medical first year students. *Int. J. Appl. Basic Med. Res.* **2015**, *5*, 124–127. [CrossRef] [PubMed]
25. Morrison, S.; Colberg, S.R.; Parson, H.K.; Vinik, A.I. Exercise improves gait, reaction time and postural stability in older adults with type 2 diabetes and neuropathy. *J. Diabetes Complicat.* **2014**, *28*, 715–722. [CrossRef]
26. Yildirim, N.U.; Erbahçeci, F.; Ergun, N.; Pitetti, K.H.; Beets, M.W. The effect of physical fitness training on reaction time in youth with intellectual disabilities. *Percept. Mot. Ski.* **2010**, *111*, 178–186. [CrossRef]
27. Della, V.E.; Palermi, S.; Aloe, I.; Marcantonio, R.; Spera, R.; Montagnani, S.; Sirico, F. Effectiveness of Workplace Yoga Interventions to Reduce Perceived Stress in Employees: A Systematic Review and Meta-Analysis. *J. Funct. Morphol. Kinesiol.* **2020**, *5*, 33. [CrossRef]
28. Yaribeygi, H.; Panahi, Y.; Sahraei, H.; Johnston, T.P.; Sahebkar, A. The impact of stress on body function: A review. *EXCLI J.* **2017**, *16*, 1057–1072.
29. O'Hagan, A.D.; Issartel, J.; McGinley, E.; Warrington, G. A pilot study exploring the effects of sleep deprivation on analogue measures of pilot competencies. *Aerosp. Med. Hum. Perform.* **2018**, *89*, 609–615. [CrossRef]
30. Baayen, R.H.; Milin, P. Analyzing reaction times. *Int. J. Psychol. Res.* **2010**, *3*, 1–27.

31. Boot, W.R.; Simons, D.J.; Stothart, C.; Stutts, C. The pervasive problem with placebos in psychology: Why active control groups are not sufficient to rule out placebo effects. *Perspect. Psychol. Sci.* **2013**, *8*, 445–454. [CrossRef] [PubMed]
32. Nuri, L.; Shadmehr, A.; Ghotbi, N.; Moghadam, A.B. Reaction time and anticipatory skill of athletes in open and closed skill-dominated sport. *Eur. J. Sport Sci.* **2013**, *13*, 431–436. [CrossRef] [PubMed]
33. Colonius, H.; Diederich, A. The optimal time window of visual-auditory integration: A reaction time analysis. *Front. Integr. Neurosci.* **2010**, *4*, 11. [CrossRef] [PubMed]

Publisher's Note: MDPI stays neutral with regard to jurisdictional claims in published maps and institutional affiliations.

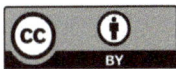 © 2020 by the authors. Licensee MDPI, Basel, Switzerland. This article is an open access article distributed under the terms and conditions of the Creative Commons Attribution (CC BY) license (http://creativecommons.org/licenses/by/4.0/).

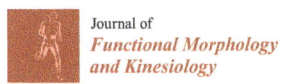

Brief Report

Differences in Balance Ability and Motor Control between Dancers and Non-Dancers with Varying Foot Positions

Brooke V. Harmon [†], Andrea N. Reed [†], Rebecca R. Rogers, Mallory R. Marshall, Joseph A. Pederson, Tyler D. Williams and Christopher G. Ballmann *

Department of Kinesiology, Samford University, 800 Lakeshore Dr., Birmingham, AL 35229, USA; bharmon@samford.edu (B.V.H.); areed2@samford.edu (A.N.R.); rrogers1@samford.edu (R.R.R.); mmarshal@samford.edu (M.R.M.); jpederso@samford.edu (J.A.P.); twilli11@samford.edu (T.D.W.)
* Correspondence: cballman@samford.edu
† These authors contributed equally.

Received: 9 June 2020; Accepted: 15 July 2020; Published: 20 July 2020

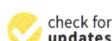

Abstract: The purpose of this study was to investigate balance and motor control in dancers and non-dancers with different foot positions. Physically active female dancers ($n = 11$) and non-dancers ($n = 9$) randomly completed two balance tests in a single visit: 1) Y-balance test (YBT), and 2) motor control test (MCT). Each test was completed with two different foot positions: 1) first ballet position in which heels were touching and feet were externally rotated to 140 degrees, and 2) sixth ballet position in which heels were spaced 10 cm apart and forward parallel. For the YBT, participants completed three attempts at anterior, posteromedial, and posterolateral reaches, which were averaged and standardized to limb length for a composite score. For the MCT, participants completed a multi-directional target test on a Biosway balance system, and accuracy and time to completion were analyzed. Findings revealed no differences in YBT score ($p = 0.255$), MCT score ($p = 0.383$), or MCT time ($p = 0.306$) between groups in the sixth position. However, dancers displayed better YBT scores ($p = 0.036$), MCT scores ($p = 0.020$), and faster MCT times ($p = 0.009$) in the first position. Results suggest that superior balance and motor control in dancers may be limited to less innate dance-specific foot positions.

Keywords: motor control test; stability; Y balance test; first position

1. Introduction

Balance, specifically human balance, is the state of the body in equilibrium with forces acting on it, which allows for the ability not to fall [1]. Different domains of balance may be under static conditions in which center of gravity (CoG) is preserved or during dynamic conditions where equilibrium must be maintained while in motion under a base support [2]. Balance ability may determine performance in highly coordinated sports (i.e., gymnastics/dance, alpine skiing, figure skating) but also predict injury risk, especially in lower extremities [3]. The sport of dance is widely accepted as necessitating balance skill, and balance exercises are highly integrated into training regimens of almost all types of dance. While static balance and stability have generally been shown to be superior in dancers compared to non-dancers, less is known about how balance control differs between them, especially in differing foot positions.

Fitness in dance is unique and primarily requires high levels of coordination and stability control. Interestingly, professional dancers have been reported to have comparable cardiorespiratory fitness to healthy sedentary counterparts despite extensive training and years of dance experience [4]. However, dancers have repeatedly been shown to have better abilities in maintaining different aspects of balance compared to non-dancers. Krtyakiarana et al. showed that classical dancers maintain postural stability to a greater degree than non-dancers, and this difference is accentuated under multitasking conditions [5]. Kilroy et al. reported dancers were able to balance for a longer period of time in a single-legged static stance on both dominant and non-dominant lower extremities [6]. Improvements in stability may be due to higher strength in plantar and hallux flexors when challenged in the anterior–posterior direction [7]. Additionally, hip strength and flexibility have been postulated as potential mechanisms of superior balance in dancers [8].

Assessments of various aspects of balance in dancers have been measured in postural (i.e., CoG), static (i.e., balance error scoring system, single leg stance on force platform), and dynamic (i.e., star excursion balance test, YBT, multiaxial stability index) aspects. Since different forms of dance have distinctive demands, using such tests to evaluate training to improve specific aspects of balance are used by dance athletes and practitioners. Dowse et al. showed improved dynamic balance assessed via multiaxial stability index and lower body strength in dancers undergoing a nine-week resistance training program [9]. Importantly, these improvements accompanied better subjective dance technique, spatial skills, and overall dance performance. Furthermore, proprioceptive–neuromuscular training regimens have been shown to improve single legged static and dynamic balance measures [10]. However, balance tests may also be used a tool to assess or predict injury risk in dancers. Filpa et al. reported that star excursion balance scores predicted function turn out angle and have been used as a marker for lower injury risk [11]. Furthermore, injured dancers have been shown to perform poorer on postural stability tests compared to uninjured dancers [12]. Thus, assessment of balance in dancers has value from a performance and health perspective.

Dance as a sport and artform has distinct physical demands highly reliant on the ability to maintain balance in a variety of different conditions. From a practical standpoint, balance ability may be able to be used to detect risk of injury, thus potentially allowing for information on personalized rehabilitation [13]. To date, most investigations have focused on static and postural stability in dancers and non-dancers in neutral foot positions. Casabona et al. reported that dancers have improved static balance in more difficult dance-specific stances, while dancers and non-dancers had similar performance in more natural foot positions [14]. However, dancing requires various foot positions with motor control and dynamic balance. Thus, understanding the multi-faceted aspects of balance adaptations in dance may provide new insight into mechanisms of training and injury risk assessment. The purpose of this study was to investigate dynamic balance ability and motor control in dancers and non-dancers in the first and sixth ballet positions.

2. Materials and Methods

2.1. Study Design

In a static groups comparison design, dancers and non-dancers randomly completed two balance tests in a single visit: 1) Y-balance test (YBT), and 2) motor control test (MCT). Each balance test was completed in a modified 1st ballet position (turned out) and 6th ballet position (parallel), which are fundamental ballet foot positions, as previously described by Casabona et al. [14]. For the 1st ballet position, heels were touching, and feet were externally rotated 140 degrees from hallux to hallux (if unipedal, the single foot was rotated 70 degrees). Visual representation of the foot positions can be seen in Figure 1. The YBT was used as a unipedal measure of dynamic balance while the MCT was a bipedal measure of multidirectional motor control. All balance tests were conducted barefoot and by the same two researchers for all measurements.

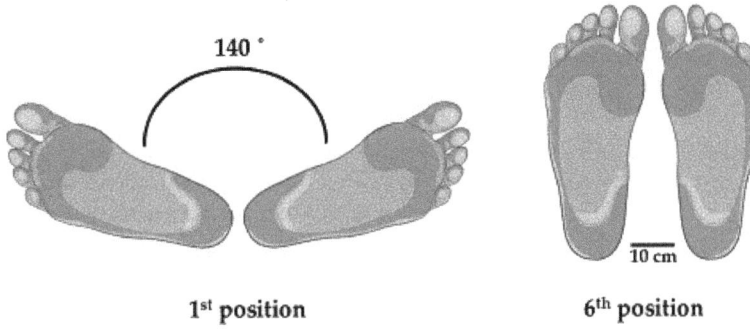

Figure 1. Visual depiction of both 6th and 1st positions used during balance tests. Note: if unipedal, the participant's single foot serving as the base was still at the same position as shown above as the sole base of support.

2.2. Participants

Physically active female dancers ($n = 11$) and non-dancers ($n = 9$) were recruited for this study. Descriptive characteristics of participants are presented in Table 1. Physically active was defined as participating in ≥150 min·wk^{-1} of moderate intensity exercise. To be categorized as a dancer, individuals had to have at least 8 years of dance experience in performance or classes (avg dance experience = 15.3 yr ± 2.06) and be actively dancing at the time of the investigation. To determine suitability for exercise, a physical activity readiness questionnaire (PARQ) was used. All participants reported no lower extremity, lumbopelvic, or musculoskeletal injury and no vestibular or balance impairments. All experimental procedures were conducted in accordance with the Declaration of Helsinki and approved by the Samford University Institutional Review Board (EXPD-HP-20-S-3).

Table 1. Descriptive characteristics of participants. * indicated significantly different from non-dancer ($p < 0.05$). Data are presented as mean ± SD.

Characteristic	Non-Dancer ($n = 9$)	Dancer ($n = 11$)
Age (yr)	19.5 ± 0.8	21.2 ± 0.7 *
Height (cm)	163.2 ± 3.9	165.3 ± 3.9
Body mass (kg)	64.3 ± 8.1	58.1 ± 6.3 *
Lower limb length (cm)	88.2 ± 4.54	85.9 ± 4.8

2.3. Y-balance Test (YBT)

The YBT is a unipedal functional test of dynamic balance. To account for possible differences in limb length, each participant's limb length (LL) of both left and right lower extremities was measured. To achieve this, participants laid supine and total length in centimeters from the anterior superior iliac spine to the distal edge of the medial malleolus was documented. A Y-balance system (Functional Movement Systems, Lynchburg, VA, USA) consisting of a central platform and three branching tubes marked in $\frac{1}{2}$ cm increments in the anterior, posteromedial, and posterolateral was utilized. On each tube, a sliding indicator block was attached to indicate reach distance during the test. Participants stood in a unipedal stance in corresponding foot positions and performed a maximal reach in each direction while moving the sliding indicator with their toes. The distance reached was recorded to the nearest $\frac{1}{2}$ cm at the proximal edge of the sliding indicator. Participants completed three successful reaches in each direction for both the left and right legs. All reaches were averaged to give a single score in each direction. A successful reach was indicated by an attempt without 1) losing balance during the extension motion and return to the platform, 2) lifting their heel off the contact foot from the platform, 3) losing contact between the reach foot and indicator, and 4) using the indicator as support/putting weight on the indicator [15]. Scores for each leg for both positions were calculated by the following calculation: ((avg anterior + avg posteromedial + avg posterolateral)/(3 × LL) × 100) [15]. Left and right leg scores were then averaged to give a total composite score for 1st and 6th ballet positions.

2.4. Biosway Motor Control Test (MCT)

To test motor and balance control, participants completed an MCT protocol on a Biosway portable balance system (Biodex Medical Systems Inc., Shirley, NY, USA) according to the manufacturer's instructions. In a bipedal stance, participants stood on a balance platform while looking at a screen display with a center point (representing CoG) and eight surrounding targets arranged in a circle. Once the test began, participants shifted and controlled their balance with their feet stationary to hit a randomly blinking target. Once the target was hit, participants had to return their balance back to the center point before another target would be highlighted. This was completed for a single test until each of the 8 targets during the attempt were hit. Participants did this once with the 1st and again with the 6th ballet position. Accuracy, or amount of deviation from the direct path to the target, and time to completion of the test were derived and recorded from the Biosway system.

2.5. Data analysis

All data was analyzed using Jamovi software (Version 0.9, Jamovie, Sydney, Australia). Normality of distribution was confirmed using a Shapiro–Wilk test. The comparison of interest was the between groups effect (i.e., dancers versus non-dancers) for each separate foot position. Thus, an independent t-test was used to compare measures between groups for each position. Cohen's d effect sizes (d) were calculated as $d = (M_1 - M_2)/(SD_{pooled})$ between groups and interpreted as 0.2—small; 0.5—moderate; and 0.8—large [16,17]. Significance was set at $p \leq 0.05$ a priori. All data were presented as mean ± standard deviation (SD).

3. Results

Descriptive characteristics are shown in Table 1. Age (years; $p < 0.001$; $d = 2.27$) was significantly higher and body mass (kg; $p = 0.012$; $d = 1.24$) lower in the dance group compared to non-dancers. No differences existed for height (cm; $p = 0.271$; $d = 0.53$) or lower limb length (cm; $p = 0.178$; $d = 0.63$). YBT composite scores are shown in Figure 2a. Participants in the dancer group scored significantly higher on the YBT compared to non-dancers when standing in the 1st ballet position (non-dancers = 83.7% ± 5.8, dancers = 90.8% ± 7.7; $p = 0.036$; $d = 1.2$). However, no differences in YBT scores were observed between groups when standing in the sixth ballet position (non-dancers = 88.8% ± 6.1, dancers = 92.4% ± 7.3; $p = 0.535$; $d = 0.2$).

MCT scores and completion times are shown in Figures 2b and 2c, respectively. Dancers scored significantly better than non-dancers on the MCT while standing in the 1st ballet position (non-dancers = 0.38 a.u. ± 0.06, dancers = 0.47 a.u. ± 0.06; $p = 0.020$; $d = 1.5$). MCT scores were not significantly different between dancers and non-dancers when standing in the sixth ballet position (non-dancers = 0.51 a.u. ± 0.06, dancers = 0.54 a.u. ± 0.04; $p = 0.383$; $d = 0.5$). MCT time to completion was significantly faster in the dancer group while standing in the 1st position (non-dancers = 34.3 s ± 4.9, dancers = 43.6 s ± 6.9; $p = 0.016$; $d = 1.5$). However, no significant difference for MCT times existed between dancers and non-dancers in the sixth ballet position (non-dancers = 36.7 s ± 7.1, dancers = 33.7 s ± 2.8; $p = 0.306$; $d = 0.5$).

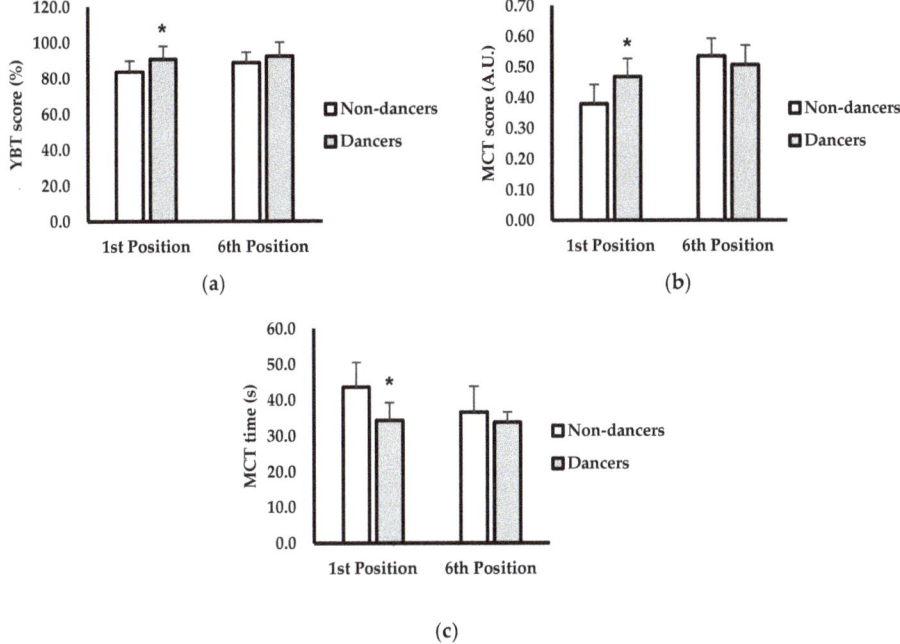

Figure 2. (a) Composite Y-balance test (YBT) scores (%) in 1st ballet position and 6th ballet position between non-dancers (white) and dancers (grey); (b) Biosway motor control test (MCT) scores (arbitrary units, A.U.) in 1st ballet position and 6th ballet position between non-dancers (white) and dancers (grey); (c) MCT completion time (s) in 1st ballet position and 6th ballet position between non-dancers (white) and dancers (grey); data are presented as mean ± SD. * Indicates significantly different from 1st position non-dancer ($p < 0.05$).

4. Discussion

While previous studies have described superior dynamic balance in dancers [18], information on how varying foot positions influence balance ability is lacking. Findings from this investigation showed no differences in dynamic balance or motor control when standing in the parallel sixth ballet position. However, dancers showed superior dynamic balance performance and motor control while standing in the turned-out first ballet position. While exact mechanisms for adaptations were not currently elucidated, these data add interesting evidence to the body of literature suggesting that dancers' superior balance and motor control performance may be limited to more dance-specific foot positions.

In the current investigation, dancers and non-dancers performed similarly on the YBT and MCT while standing in the sixth ballet position. This is in stark contrast to previous findings, which have largely shown dancers to have better balance in similar neutral foot positions. Kilroy et al. reported that dancers were able to balance longer and maintain CoG to a greater degree in a unipedal stance compared to non-dancers [6]. However, Kilroy et al. utilized static balance measurements through a force platform, which differed from the unipedal dynamic approach in the current study. Static and dynamic balance require different levels of joint stabilization and abilities to produce muscular force [19]. While joint stiffness and co-contracture of muscles may be important for static balance, weak relationships for stiffness and adaptations often leading to improvements in dynamic balance (i.e., strength, muscle force, etc.) have been reported previously [20]. Since adaptations with dance training may manifest themselves in increased joint stability and stiffness [21], dance training may have a greater impact on unipedal static versus unipedal dynamic balance in neutral foot positions. Supporting this, Ambegaonkar et al. reported that unipedal static stability was higher in dancers versus non-dancers, but balance did not differ in alternating leg dynamic tests and only differed in a portion of directions for dynamic reach tests [22]. In contrast, there have been previous investigations showing superior dynamic balance in young dancers versus non-dancers, necessitating more study for what mechanisms are underlying balance adaptations to static and dynamic conditions differently [18]. Another possible explanation for lack of difference in the sixth position may be due to the familiarity of the position in that most able-bodied individuals will likely stand with feet pointed parallel on a daily basis. Indeed, Casabona et al. reported that more natural neutral foot positions did not alter static balance outcomes in dancers versus non-dancers, while more challenging dance-specific stances caused dancers to perform better [14]. Our findings of no changes in dynamic measures or motor control using natural stances supports this, although there have been other investigations showing better dynamic balance in dancers versus non-dancers with neutral foot positions [18,23]. However, participants in the non-dancer group in the current investigation were still considered physically active. Higher levels of physical activity, both free-living and structured, have been shown to improve balance outcomes [24,25]. Thus, training habits of the non-dancers may have resulted in similar adaptations to dancers, which allowed for similar balance and control in the sixth position. However, differences in regular training habits of dancer and non-dancer groups was not investigated in the current study, leaving the contribution of specific aspects of exercise training unclear. Based on this, future investigations should attempt to delineate specific fitness measures and how they correspond to balance and motor control differently in dancers and non-dancers.

Despite lack of differences in the sixth position, dancers displayed better dynamic balance in the YBT and better motor control in the MCT while standing in the first position. These findings are supported by Casabona et al. who showed that dancers exhibited better static balance while standing in an identical turned out position as the present study but not in neutral positions [14]. Likely, differences between dancers and non-dancers are due to training specificity. Balancing while externally rotated requires high levels of hip and ankle strength and flexibility. Indeed, Gupta et al. showed that dancers have greater hip strength and range of motion compared to non-dancers [8]. Additionally, while individual motor skills may have certain degrees of transferability to others, extensive practice and training may result in more specialized capabilities, which lead to adaptation in the trained skill that may not be generalizable [14,26]. In relation to the current findings, extensive practice in dancers may have led to particularly improved skill in the first position, which is largely a dance-specific skill that did not transfer to superior balance in the sixth position. Important to the current investigation, dancers were more accurate and faster during the MCT compared to non-dancers. This suggests that dancers not only displayed more effective multi-directional balance control but could do so more efficiently. These findings may have practical implications for predicting injury risk. Previous evidence in basketball players reported multi-directional balance performance was predictive of lower extremity injury risk [27]. Furthermore, athletes with higher balance ability before starting the competition season have been shown to be less likely to be injured during the season [28]. While largely speculative based off the current study design, using accuracy and time of motor control tests in various positions in dance could possibly lead to prediction of which foot positions during dance performance may lead to higher rates of injuries in individuals. Supporting this, reduced functional turnout angles in the first ballet position have been shown to be associated with higher numbers and severity of injury in professional dancers [29]. However, injury risk was not measured in the current investigation but could be a practical application for subsequent studies to investigate.

5. Conclusions

The current brief report provides novel evidence on balance and motor control between dancers and non-dancers. However, there were several limitations. Although the sample size of the current investigation is in agreement with similar studies [6,14], large samples are warranted in order to maximize generalizability and comparison to other dance populations. Anthropometric features (i.e., body mass, body composition, etc.) were not controlled between groups, and dancers in the present study tended to be lighter than non-dancers. However, sports like dance and gymnastics have been consistently documented to have a tendency of smaller athletes [30]. Total body and lean mass has been shown to influence balance ability; thus, we cannot rule out the possibility of body composition affecting the results [31]. Furthermore, very recent evidence has shown that YBT performance may be related to trunk and lower limb strength [32]. Unfortunately, this specific information was not obtained with the current study design, so present YBT results should be viewed with optimism but also caution. More study is needed to investigate body characteristic differences between dancers and non-dancers and how they may specially alter balance and motor control ability. Additionally, no adaptive mechanisms possibly contributing to changes in balance performance were measured. Given that numerous factors including proprioception, flexibility, and muscular strength may predict balance ability [7,33], more specific study on which factors may contribute to changes in performance with different foot positions is needed. In conclusion, dance participation and experience may not influence balance and motor control in the sixth ballet position but result in better balance outcomes while standing in the first ballet position. These findings provide new information pertaining to functional performance in dancers and may have implications for identifying specific training adaptations and injury risk in varying foot positions.

Author Contributions: Conceptualization, B.V.H., A.N.R., R.R.R., M.R.M, J.A.P., T.D.W., C.G.B.; methodology, B.V.H., A.N.R., R.R.R., M.R.M., J.A.P., T.D.W., C.G.B.; formal analysis, C.G.B.; investigation, B.V.H., A.N.R., R.R.R., M.R.M., J.A.P., T.D.W., C.G.B.; data curation, B.V.H., A.N.R., C.G.B.; writing—original draft preparation, B.V.H., A.N.R., C.G.B.; writing—review and editing, R.R.R., M.R.M., J.A.P., T.D.W., C.G.B.; supervision, R.R.R., C.G.B.; project administration, C.G.B.; All authors have read and agreed to the published version of the manuscript.

Funding: This research received no external funding

Acknowledgments: The authors would like to thank John Petrella for his support with this project.

Conflicts of Interest: The authors declare no conflict of interest.

References

1. Pollock, A.S.; Durward, B.R.; Rowe, P.J.; Paul, J.P. What is balance? *Clin. Rehabil.* **2000**, *14*, 402–406. [CrossRef] [PubMed]
2. Patton, J.L.; Pai, Y.-C.; Lee, W.A. Evaluation of a model that determines the stability limits of dynamic balance. *Gait Posture* **1999**, *9*, 38–49. [CrossRef]
3. Hrysomallis, C. Balance ability and athletic performance. *Sports Med.* **2011**, *41*, 221–232. [CrossRef] [PubMed]
4. Koutedakis, Y.; Jamurtas, A. The dancer as a performing athlete: Physiological considerations. *Med. Probl. Perform. Artist.* **2005**, *20*, 109–111. [CrossRef]
5. Krityakiarana, W.; Jongkamonwiwat, N. Comparison of balance performance between Thai classical dancers and non-dancers. *J. Dance Med. Sci.* **2016**, *20*, 72–78. [CrossRef] [PubMed]
6. Kilroy, E.A.; Crabtree, O.M.; Crosby, B.; Parker, A.; Barfield, W.R. The effect of single-leg stance on dancer and control group static balance. *Int. J. Exerc. Sci.* **2016**, *9*, 110.
7. Rowley, K.M.; Jarvis, D.N.; Kurihara, T.; Chang, Y.-J.; Fietzer, A.L.; Kulig, K. Toe flexor strength, flexibility and function and flexor hallucis longus tendon morphology in dancers and non-dancers. *Med. Probl. Perform. Artist.* **2015**, *30*, 152–156. [CrossRef] [PubMed]
8. Gupta, A.; Fernihough, B.; Bailey, G.; Bombeck, P.; Clarke, A.; Hopper, D. An evaluation of differences in hip external rotation strength and range of motion between female dancers and non-dancers. *Br. J. Sports Med.* **2004**, *38*, 778–783. [CrossRef] [PubMed]
9. Dowse, R.A.; McGuigan, M.R.; Harrison, C. Effects of a resistance training intervention on strength, power, and performance in adolescent dancers. *J. Strength Cond. Res.* **2017**. [CrossRef] [PubMed]
10. Tekin, D.; Agopyan, A.; Baltaci, G. Balance training in modern dancers: Proprioceptive-neuromuscular training vs kinesio taping. *Med. Probl. Perform. Artist.* **2018**, *33*, 156–165. [CrossRef]
11. Filipa, A.R.; Smith, T.R.; Paterno, M.V.; Ford, K.R.; Hewett, T.E. Performance on the Star Excursion Balance Test predicts functional turnout angle in pre-pubescent female dancers. *J. Dance Med. Sci.* **2013**, *17*, 165–169. [CrossRef] [PubMed]
12. Lin, C.-F.; Lee, I.-J.; Liao, J.-H.; Wu, H.-W.; Su, F.-C. Comparison of postural stability between injured and uninjured ballet dancers. *Am. J. Sports Med.* **2011**, *39*, 1324–1331. [CrossRef]

13. Clark, T.; Redding, E. The relationship between postural stability and dancer's past and future lower-limb injuries. *Med. Probl. Perform. Artist.* **2012**, *27*, 197. [CrossRef]
14. Casabona, A.; Leonardi, G.; Aimola, E.; La Grua, G.; Polizzi, C.M.; Cioni, M.; Valle, M.S. Specificity of foot configuration during bipedal stance in ballet dancers. *Gait Posture* **2016**, *46*, 91–97. [CrossRef] [PubMed]
15. Gonell, A.C.; Romero, J.A.P.; Soler, L.M. Relationship between the Y balance test scores and soft tissue injury incidence in a soccer team. *Int. J. Sports Phys. Ther.* **2015**, *10*, 955.
16. Fritz, C.O.; Morris, P.E.; Richler, J.J. Effect size estimates: Current use, calculations, and interpretation. *J. Exp. Psychol. Gen.* **2012**, *141*, 2–18. [CrossRef] [PubMed]
17. Cohen, J. *Statistical Power Analysis for the Behavioral Sciences*, 2nd ed.; Lawrence Erlbaum Associates: Hillsdale, NJ, USA, 1988.
18. Da Silveira Costa, M.S.; de Sá Ferreira, A.; Felicio, L.R. Static and dynamic balance in ballet dancers: A literature review. *Fisioter. Pesqui* **2013**, *20*, 299–305.
19. Çelenk, Ç.; Marangoz, İ.; Aktuğ, Z.B.; Top, E.; Akıl, M. The effect of quadriceps femoris and hamstring muscular force on static and dynamic balance performance. *Int. J. Phys. Educ. Sports Health* **2015**, *2*, 323–325.
20. Owen, G.; Cronin, J.; Gill, N.; McNair, P. Knee extensor stiffness and functional performance. *Phys. Ther. Sport* **2005**, *6*, 38–44. [CrossRef]
21. Phillips, C. Stability in dance training. *J. Dance Med. Sci.* **2005**, *9*, 24–28.
22. Ambegaonkar, J.P.; Caswell, S.V.; Winchester, J.B.; Shimokochi, Y.; Cortes, N.; Caswell, A.M. Balance comparisons between female dancers and active nondancers. *Res. Q. Exerc. Sport* **2013**, *84*, 24–29. [CrossRef]
23. Golomer, E.; Dupui, P.; Séréni, P.; Monod, H. The contribution of vision in dynamic spontaneous sways of male classical dancers according to student or professional level. *J. Physiol. Paris* **1999**, *93*, 233–237. [CrossRef]
24. Iwakura, M.; Okura, K.; Shibata, K.; Kawagoshi, A.; Sugawara, K.; Takahashi, H.; Shioya, T. Relationship between balance and physical activity measured by an activity monitor in elderly COPD patients. *Int. J. Chronic Obstr. Pulm. Dis.* **2016**, *11*, 1505. [CrossRef] [PubMed]
25. Ferreira, M.L.; Sherrington, C.; Smith, K.; Carswell, P.; Bell, R.; Bell, M.; Nascimento, D.P.; Pereira, L.S.M.; Vardon, P. Physical activity improves strength, balance and endurance in adults aged 40–65 years: A systematic review. *J. Physiother.* **2012**, *58*, 145–156. [CrossRef]
26. Keetch, K.M.; Schmidt, R.A.; Lee, T.D.; Young, D.E. Especial skills: Their emergence with massive amounts of practice. *J. Exp. Psychol. Hum. Percept. Perform.* **2005**, *31*, 970. [CrossRef] [PubMed]
27. Plisky, P.J.; Rauh, M.J.; Kaminski, T.W.; Underwood, F.B. Star Excursion Balance Test as a predictor of lower extremity injury in high school basketball players. *J. Orthop. Sports Phys. Ther.* **2006**, *36*, 911–919. [CrossRef]
28. Olivier, B.; Stewart, A.; Olorunju, S.; McKinon, W. Static and dynamic balance ability, lumbo-pelvic movement control and injury incidence in cricket pace bowlers. *J. Sci. Med. Sport* **2015**, *18*, 19–25. [CrossRef]
29. Negus, V.; Hopper, D.; Briffa, N.K. Associations between turnout and lower extremity injuries in classical ballet dancers. *J. Orthop. Sports Phys. Ther.* **2005**, *35*, 307–318. [CrossRef]
30. Norton, K.; Olds, T.; Olive, S.; Craig, N. Anthropometry and sports performance. In *Anthropometrica: A Textbook of Body Measurement for Sports and Health Courses*; Norton, K., Olds, T., Eds.; UNSW Press: Radwick, Australia, 1996; pp. 287–364.
31. Handrigan, G.; Hue, O.; Simoneau, M.; Corbeil, P.; Marceau, P.; Marceau, S.; Tremblay, A.; Teasdale, N. Weight loss and muscular strength affect static balance control. *Int. J. Obes.* **2010**, *34*, 936–942. [CrossRef] [PubMed]
32. Fusco, A.; Giancotti, G.F.; Fuchs, P.X.; Wagner, H.; da Silva, R.A.; Cortis, C. Y balance test: Are we doing it right? *J. Sci. Med. Sport* **2020**, *23*, 194–199. [CrossRef]
33. Ambegaonkar, J.P.; Mettinger, L.M.; Caswell, S.V.; Burtt, A.; Cortes, N. Relationships between core endurance, hip strength, and balance in collegiate female athletes. *Int. J. Sports Phys. Ther.* **2014**, *9*, 604. [PubMed]

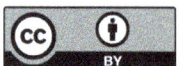

© 2020 by the authors. Licensee MDPI, Basel, Switzerland. This article is an open access article distributed under the terms and conditions of the Creative Commons Attribution (CC BY) license (http://creativecommons.org/licenses/by/4.0/).

MDPI
St. Alban-Anlage 66
4052 Basel
Switzerland
Tel. +41 61 683 77 34
Fax +41 61 302 89 18
www.mdpi.com

Journal of Functional Morphology and Kinesiology Editorial Office
E-mail: jfmk@mdpi.com
www.mdpi.com/journal/jfmk

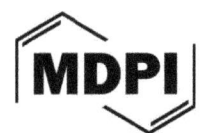

www.ingramcontent.com/pod-product-compliance
Lightning Source LLC
LaVergne TN
LVHW070045120526
838202LV00101B/630